caring for somebody with dementia

Merideth Sindel

connorcourt
PUBLISHING

Connor Court Publishing Pty Ltd.
PO Box 1
Ballan VIC 3342
sales@connorcourt.com
www.connorcourt.com

ISBN: 9781921421754 (pbk.)

Front cover design: Ian James

Printed and designed in Australia.

Back cover photo: Merideth Sindel as a child with her mother.

For my sister,

for her inspiration and practical sense.

Contents

Preface

Nobody expects their parent to get dementia. Until her eightieth birthday everybody thought my mother was as sharp as a tack. There were some problems, of course there were. She had never fully recovered from a hip replacement that had gone badly. She was slowing down and that irritated her though her determination remained the same. But within a handful of years her dementia was obvious.

It had been slow-growing. It took some years to build up a head of steam. It would leap out sometimes to give me cause for concern and then tuck itself away again.

Mum had only ever helped people. She had spent her life helping people. She had always been *there for you.* So practical. Vital. The most reliable person you'd know. But then the eyes started changing and she became prone to rages. She would be making endless lists of things and discussing the lists until you felt your brain was going to mollify and leak out through the ears. How much money should go in the bills tin, how much dinner the cat should get! On and on it went. I remember when the Census forms came and she made a complete botch of them, *again.* Oh, yes, the word dementia had crept into my head more than once.

In 2001 my brother died and it did not register with Mum in any normal fashion. I was getting surer.

After that she began conjuring up dead relatives. 'We haven't had Uncle Harry over to lunch for a while. I've been remiss. I should do something about that.'

Then she would remember and wonder at herself. 'Harry's dead, of course! I must be going *senile!*'

'Don't worry, Mum. You're fine,' I would say, stabs of electricity going down my spine.

Of course she wasn't fine. One day she fainted en route to the supermarket and another time she fell and broke her pelvis. It was then that the cat crept out of its bag.

She was in hospital for six weeks then, two weeks in the ward and a month in rehab. And it was then that it became obvious. From her hospital bed she was saying such things as: 'Brian came to see me last night. He's looking very thin. He could do with some fattening up!' Brian, my father, had been dead for nearly twenty years.

I know rehab can be long and depressing, but the problems were obvious. When Mum came home from hospital and delusions and hallucinations started blazing their way through our house I went to the GP for help and he did urine and blood tests to rule out infection. But there was no infection. And so it had become obvious.

By then I had left my nine to five job and was free to slip into the role of looking after her. I took over the reigns. They were shaking in my hands, but after some years of turmoil everything calmed down. I looked after her then. Mum knew I looked after her then and everything became easier. In some ways we went back to *normal*.

But nobody expects that their parent will get dementia, nobody is prepared for it, and in the beginning I had no real understanding, no real idea of what to expect. I was primed for horrors by the stereotypical images on television. Though I had worked in a hospital for ten years and had seen second-hand the effects of dementia, I still had no real understanding of it. Memory loss, I figured. Disappearance. Apart from that I was absolutely clueless. I even looked up on the internet: 'clothes for people with dementia'. That's how bewildered I was.

Mum was having bad delusions – thinking home was somewhere else. What do you do? What do you say when your mother wants to start packing in readiness for going home when you're already home? Do you put select possessions in boxes and drive around the block? Is there a standard response to these problems?

I phoned the Dementia Helpline hoping for some immediate

advice.

'Is it an emergency?' the person said. She took my number and said somebody would phone back.

A couple of days later I was offered a place in an eight-week course on caring for somebody with memory loss and dementia. The course was due to begin in March, which was weeks away. Mum could go to a coping with memory loss group while I attended the dementia course.

The operator asked how I coped, what was I doing in response to the delusions. I said I had started 'delaying and distracting', something I had read on the internet. ('Delaying' I supposed meant putting off 'going home' until another time, and 'distracting' I supposed meant doing something else.) That's the way to go, the person said.

I told Mum about the courses, but she was only affronted: 'There's nothing wrong with my memory. I can remember my days from primary school!' And of course she could.

I decided then I was going to have to figure this out myself. You are going to have to work it out as you go along, I told myself. And that is what I have done. This book shows how I coped and at times didn't cope at all. What I learnt along the way is that there are no hard and fast rules for dealing with such horrors as delusions; there are only things you can try. And calm and cheerfulness goes a long way to keeping the person happy.

In fact as time went on I just dismissed much of the advice I had read in those early days:

Avoid shopping centres and other crowded places. Mum loved shopping centres. She enjoyed the activity and being 'where the people are'.

Don't take her on holiday. We did travel once and had the opportunity arisen I'd have done it again. Mum was fine.

Don't announce changes or plans in advance. It's true, there would be the endless questions and sometimes worrying. But having plans gave Mum something to look forward to and scheme over. If I announced plans or changes in advance she felt included.

Don't just *take over*. **If you are taking over when the person would rather choose their own clothes, for example, you may cause anger and frustration without even understanding why.** But for us it was not long before I found it was easier if I just helped with such things as dressing. Offering too many choices – 'Which dress, Mum? The red? The green? Or would you like your slacks with the nice top?' – can be an unnecessary source of confusion in itself. I took over everything for Mum and that worked for us. I accept that it does not work for everybody.

Beware of sundowning. Sundowning is the expected spike in confusion that can come in the afternoon or evening. One theory behind sundowning is that people with dementia expend so much energy trying to make sense of their world that by the afternoon they are mentally exhausted. But what difference does it make? People are all different and those of us with dementia do not necessarily follow the guidelines. The advice on sundowning was: **Don't plan activities for the afternoons or 'sundowning' time.** Now I would say, are you crazy? Mum was happier if she was busy. It did not matter what time of the day it was. Going out in the afternoons or having some other activity to focus on actually staved off delusions.

I started looking after Mum September 2002. I was expecting the illness to claim her within a matter of months. That's how bad she seemed to me then. In the end I wanted our life together to just go on and on. But, of course, it wasn't going to go on and on, and she died in early January 2006. Three years. Three years and four months to be exact.

For all that time Dementia sat himself between us – or at least he tried to. He was a spiteful fellow and had brought with him his hideous companions, delusions, anxiety, depression. He sat there trying to cast shadows between us, though often enough I could elbow him out of the road. I knew she was still there.

It can be easy to overlook the person with dementia. The words may not come in a hurry any more. The exception to that rule for Mum was when she was angry with me. Then the words flowed easily enough!

When she was quiet people might talk about her or over her as if she couldn't hear any more. She could still hear! Actually, sometimes I thought the quietness suited her purpose. It was easier than having to try and find the words, but that didn't mean she could not understand. She understood. There were even times when I wondered if Mum kept her real thoughts to herself, that the things she simply did not wish to disclose remained hidden.

Other times I saw her overwhelmed by Dementia. Dementia, the passionless phenomenon! Dementia, the scrawny demon! If only I could have taken him by the throat and thrown him in a corner and said 'Belt up! I need to talk to my mother about this!' and let her have her say. Are we okay, Mum? Am I doing any of it right? And she would have said: 'Of course you are, my darling!'

In many ways life with my mother over those three years was the way it used to be. There had been the hideous interim period in the build-up to all this when she was insufferable, impossible. Those were hard days. Those days were murder. It was like living with an imposter. Nobody knew what was wrong with her. But then we worked it out and everything changed when I started looking after her. I was her lambie. And, if I'm honest, she was my lambie.

'Where would I be without you?' she said sometimes, which I thought was awful. 'If I didn't have you I'd be ... in hospital or somewhere.'

'Oh, you *do* have me, don't you?' I would come back.

Some days were bad. Some days I'd have gladly handed her over to somebody else, but only for a couple of hours. Then we went back to normal. Of course it was down to me at those times to take us back to normal. When things were bad it was down to me to re-establish an atmosphere of lightness, to reintroduce some casual humour. And when I had pulled that off she would be laughing again at some aside. 'You're bold!' she would be saying again.

After three years the hours seemed longer, but I knew I was coping infinitely better than in the beginning. It hadn't been nearly as fearsome as I had expected it would be. Sometimes I would even forget she had dementia. That's how used to it I became. Sometimes I had to remind myself. The important thing was still the relationship.

I think many people didn't understand that. They didn't see how much of Mum was still there. Even after three years there was an awful lot she still knew. I think people didn't realise that. Maybe delusions had put a blind up between them and her and they didn't get to look behind it.

Every so often somebody would tell me I was wonderful. 'It's an honourable thing you do, looking after your mother like that,' they would say, as if nobody had ever thought of it before. I was no more honourable than before, certainly more assertive and more confident, but no more honourable. I was impatient many times and made many mistakes. But I still liked and loved and admired my mother more than I did others and she knew that so there was balance.

I began the Preface for this book just as Mum was getting ill. She was dying actually, though I still had hopes. And so I wrote: 'We are hurtling towards our fourth Christmas. I try not to worry so much about the future anymore. I do, of course. There's no point in it, but still I do it. I lie in bed surrounded by what ifs. What if I can't do this anymore? What if – or when – she becomes bedridden? What if I simply can't lift her anymore? Hoists and things? Maybe it's not that easy.' What if? What if? But ultimately I always went back to The Mission. *My mission now is the same as when I started – to keep her safe and happy.*' And it was comforting. It was a good mission. And so the future and all its what ifs were shelved yet again.

We were not alone, Mum and I. My sister and her family lived directly beside us. Brother-in-law Colin pumped up the tyres of the wheelchair. Nephew Alexander (Rock) fixed the television and computer when they went on the blink. Middle nephew Cameron came in for videos and chats with Grandma. He would often 'mind' her when I had to go to the bank or wherever. When we were off to the shops we often passed the youngest, Nick, on his way home from school. My sister was always there to do yackety-yak over what was happening in the world. We were not alone.

Some days were an endurance test. Sometimes I felt that all I did was walk around, from one room to the next, doing the things *I* had forgotten to do, retrieving the things Mum thought she had lost – her handbag, her glasses, her stick. Often I was fed up with the sound of my own voice – repeating myself, explaining, reassuring. And often in the middle of the day she might start to go quiet and sorrowful and that was when I had to think quickly – to place myself with a spark of an idea between her and an impending delusion.

Mum had dementia. She could be very strange some days, but I thought it didn't matter how odd she became just so long as she was happy – or happy enough – and safe.

And she was happy – or happy enough. We still talked all the time and shared a laugh. What did we talk about? Everything. Or nearly everything. In the old days her interests were theology and politics and history and she still showed appreciation at some level although, of course, it became me back-talking the commentators on the television instead of her. A lot of that was gone. The academic fervour for church history and politics, especially, had simply gone, been wiped off. But she could still tell one political leader from another. She had always mistrusted Conservatives and she still mistrusted Conservatives. She had always admired Kim Beazley and she still admired Kim Beazley. In the June 2005 Budget Mr Beazley was heading the ALP, and Mum sat glued to his reply to the Budget: 'Well done … What's his name? Kim! Well done, Kim!'

She watched the news obsessively every day and sometimes I read bits from the paper to her. She muddled some parts. One item of news was glued to the next. But she still showed interest in what was going on. When we talked about Schapelle Corby and the Bali Nine she had them muddled. And when she had things muddled her *modus operandi* was simply to dismiss one of them. Schapelle Corby rated high in her thinking, but the Bali Nine flew under the radar. I think that was the main difference. She would watch documentaries on a range of subjects, from storm chasers to statesmen, and seem to follow them well enough.

One night I was in the kitchen when she called out: 'Bob Carr has resigned!' I wondered if she had that right, but she was right. Bob Carr *had* resigned. Mum was still there.

There were hard times, of course there were. The unpleasant aspects of her character were over-accentuated. She was more worried, more nervous. She also became extremely frail. And her delusions and despairs were fierce. She couldn't remember that her mother, her husband and her eldest son were all dead and she looked and looked for them. She would have sooled Interpol onto them if only she could have located Interpol.

I didn't get much time off. That goes without saying. Mum went to a day centre on Mondays, though I knew that was coming to an end. I had never been sure about sending her there, though some days, of course, I was glad to see the back of her. And a care worker came in from Kincare – one of the government-subsidised agencies – once a week and then once a fortnight for an hour and a half. It was Lisa for two years and then Lisa decided to change jobs. I was dreading changing workers, but after Lisa we were allocated Susan who was a wonderful all-hands-to-the-pump type. She and Mum just sat together and talked and talked. That worked.

In the final year we discovered Community Transport. So then, mercifully, we were getting out more. They took us on outings into the city and once a fortnight the bus picked us up and we went to a local shopping centre. The driver left us to our own devices for two and a half hours, then picked us up and brought us home again. We had a cheeseburger, did some shopping, played with the puppies in Pet's Paradise. Community Transport is a godsend.

I was thinking of calling this book *Time Best Spent with You* because that's how I saw it. That time was best spent with Mum.

My hope is that this book puts a human face to the tragedy of the illness and opens up some of the problems that may be encountered. Looking back, I can say that caring for somebody with dementia comes down to common sense, instinct and stick-at-it-ness. Three years on there were still delusions. There were wonderful times and awful times. But I wouldn't have been doing anything else if you paid me.

> **The key to looking after somebody with dementia is acceptance. Acceptance of the change. Acceptance of your new role. Acceptance of the character of Dementia. He's cruel, even selfish. But that is his character. Nobody is going to be able to talk him down or reason him away. It's just the way he is. And you have to mould yourself to fit the new situation. Anybody who learns acceptance up front is going to be streets ahead.**

Chapter 1
Description and causes of dementia

The causes of dementia

Most of us don't get dementia. Even so, up to twenty per cent of people aged 75 have dementia. And people over 85 years are up to fifty times more likely than others to get dementia. In the scheme of things that amounts to very many people.

The causes of dementia must be simple. Sometimes I wondered if Mum had just worn herself out. But she was direct evidence against the use-it-or-lose-it theory. Mum had always used her brain. She didn't do crosswords or play scrabble, but she was always reading, projecting, analysing, studying.

Some years earlier she had had a fit while out in the city doing her voluntary work. A CT scan showed nothing, but sometimes I wonder if she sustained an injury to her brain then, or perhaps the fit was just another symptom.

Some people think the use of non-steroidal anti-inflammatory drugs (ibuprofen and asprin) may help reduce brain inflammation and therefore protect the brain against Alzheimer's. But Mum had used asprin for pain relief all her adult life and she almost certainly had Alzheimer's.

My sister used to say if only we could take out Mum's brain and give it a good wash. And that points closer to the truth. People with Alzheimer's have an accumulation of plaque called amyloid in the brain. Some researchers work on addressing the effects of the plaque. Others are working on what causes the plaque in the first place. Some are focused on the connection between stress and dementia. Others work on links with the natural draining away of testosterone and estrogen that comes with old age. Some researchers have found a connection between high blood pressure and dementia. Others still believe that people with high cholesterol may be more susceptible to dementia than others. (Mum had high cholesterol.)

Whoever is on the right track or tracks – at some time in the future there will be medication that counteracts the effects of the plaque.

Different types of dementia

The American Association of Psychiatry simply describes dementia as a brain injury. There are several different types of dementia, though the fundamental associated problems remain the same or similar.

Alzheimer's disease

Alzheimer's disease is a disease that damages the brain. Seventy per cent of dementia is caused by Alzheimer's disease. The progress of the disease is slow. Some people show changes to personality and increased irritability in the early stages. Delusions and hallucinations are common in the later stages. The diagnosis of Alzheimer's comes when other possible causes have been eliminated.

Vascular dementia

Vascular dementia is caused by one or more strokes sufficiently severe to impair brain function. The person may suffer from impaired memory function, confusion, hallucinations and delusions. Treatment for hypertension may slow the disease.

Parkinson's disease

Parkinson's disease is a neurological condition that can lead to dementia. The most recognisable feature of PD is the tremor.

Lewy body disease

People with Lewy body disease have microscopic proteins in the brain. Dementia caused by Lewy body disease is similar to Alzheimer's.

Pick's disease

Pick's disease is a rare form of frontal lobe dementia which commonly occurs in people aged between fifty and sixty. The progress of the disease is generally more rapid than Alzheimer's.

Other causes

Huntington's disease may lead to dementia. Other causes include brain injury from physical trauma, AIDS, alcohol abuse and extreme vitamin deficiency.

The list seems grim, but when you think of dementia as being caused by illness or trauma then hopefully it becomes less grim.

The tests for dementia

Basically, dementia is diagnosed when brain injury is sufficient to impact on a person's ability to think clearly enough to continue to care for themselves and be a part of society.

A brain scan tests for atrophy. The Mini Mental State Examination (MMSE) tests for understanding. The MMSE is a short list of questions and tasks that investigate awareness, language and abstract thinking. The full test can be exhaustive. Points are allocated for each correct answer. Here is a sample:

Orientation		Score	points
1. What is the:	Year?	____	1
	Season?	____	1
	Date?	____	1
	Day?	____	1
	Month?	____	1
2. Where are we?	State?	____	1
	Country?	____	1
	Town or city?	____	1
	Hospital?	____	1
	Floor? (of the hospital)	____	1

Registration

3. Name three objects, taking one second to say each. Then ask the patient to repeat all three names after you have said them. (Give one point for each correct answer.) Repeat the answers until the patient learns all three. _____ 3

Attention and calculation

4. Serial sevens. Have the patient count backwards from 100 by 7s. (Stop after five answers: 93, 86, 79, 72, 65. Give one point for each correct answer.) Alternatively, have the patient spell WORLD backwards. _____ 5

Recall

5. Ask for the names of the three objects learned in question 3. (Give one point for each correct answer.) _____ 3

Language

6. Point to a pencil and a watch. Have the patient name them as you point.

_____ 2

7. Have the patient repeat 'No ifs, ands or buts.' _____ 1

8. Have the patient follow a three-stage command: 'Take a paper in your hand. Fold the paper in half. Put the paper on the floor.' _____ 3

9. Have the patient read and obey the following: 'CLOSE YOUR EYES.' (Write the words in large letters.) _____ 1

10. Have the patient write a sentence of his or her choice. (The sentence should contain a subject and an object, and it should make sense. Ignore spelling errors when scoring.) _____ 1

11. Have the patient copy a given design. (Give one point if all sides and angles are preserved and if the intersecting sides form a quadrangle _____ 1

The stages of Alzheimer's disease

Alzheimer's disease is the most common cause of dementia and is slow-growing. A person may have the disease for years and nobody notices, or if they do notice changes, they just accept them as part of the ageing process.

Stage 1 or mild dementia

- There will be memory loss. The person may say the same thing over and over, having forgotten that they have told you this story/information already.
- They may lose things more often than expected.
- They may experience a personality change, become 'difficult', unable to accept change.
- This person may seem to be burdened by sadness/grief/ depression and lose interest in the things they once enjoyed or, more likely, feel they are not able to do the things they once enjoyed.
- They may be worried about themselves and be aware that something is amiss; that promotes anxiety and depression.
- There may be covering up and coping mechanisms. For example, they may cope by making lists of things to be remembered.

People with mild dementia may have trouble working out their own finances or keeping track of their medication. (Mum used a calendar to record her medication. She would also tip tablets out of their containers and count them to be sure she had taken the required dose. Heaven help me if I offered suggestions.)

Mum had always told the same story over and over. Now it was over and over and over and over. She also experienced major changes in personality. She had become 'territorial', easily upset, more prone to irritation, even rages.

Stage 2 or moderate dementia

- The person may get lost easily.
- They may be confused about what is happening and have over the top reactions to change and things not understood.
- They may have trouble with activities we all take for granted, such as dressing
- The person may believe that fictions are reality and take a firm stand when contradicted.
- They may have hallucinations.
- They may pace or wander.
- The person may be anxious and/or depressed.
- They may have poor judgement and think they are still capable of, for example, driving.
- They may get night hours confused with daylight hours and be up and dressed when everybody else would expect to be asleep.

A lot of this was Mum. People with moderate dementia usually need a high degree of supervision. Those with moderate impairment also have difficulties with jobs such as cooking and housework.

The moderate stage of Alzheimer's is the longest stage. It can last for ten years or longer.

Stage 3 or severe dementia

- The person may lose language.
- They may cease to recognise themselves or others.

A person with severe dementia will need constant care, including personal care, feeding and so forth. Some people with severe dementia do maintain physical mobility, but have no other skills to look after themselves.

- Be aware that you will most likely have to pay the person's bills and do the banking now.
- Make sure the person has made a will.
- A lot of people advocate taking out power of attorney, but I could not see the need for us. I was Mum's next of kin. And Mum signed over Third Party at the bank to me. The bank would allow me to sign withdrawal slips for her when she was no longer able. That was good enough for us.

'Memory' medications

Selegiline, used for the treatment of Parkinson's disease, may help slow the progress of the disease. Possible side effects include nausea, vivid dreams and low blood pressure.

Some people advocate the use of vitamin E, which lacks the side effects of other medication, but that sounds a bit like the equivalent of a medical platitude to me.

The 'memory' medications used to try and slow the advance of Alzheimer's are Aricept, Exelon, Razadyne (formerly known as Reminyl) and tacrine. They come from a class of drugs called cholinesterase-inhibitors which block the enzyme responsible for the destruction of acetylcholine, one of the neurotransmitters that allow communication inside the brain.

A geriatrician prescribes the memory medication. You can get a referral to a private geriatrician from the GP or contact the Aged Care Assessment Team (ACAT) of the local hospital to arrange a brain scan and assessment. Social workers and geriatricians will come to the house for the assessment and follow up.

It was a procedure that I never pursued. I thought about it in the beginning, but shelved it as being too hard, and kept on shelving it. Mum would have hated it. The tests would have set her right back.

Christina Bryden, who was diagnosed with fronto-temporal dementia when she was 46, swears by the medication. 'Anti-dementia drugs, such as the cholinesterase inhibitors, should be offered as soon as possible after diagnosis. They can help what remains to work better.'[1] And for a younger person you would certainly grab it with both hands.

But Mum was not a younger person and the discussion would have been one-way. Early in the peace I contacted a psychogeriatric nurse who came to the house and did the MMSE on Mum. Mum answered the questions politely, but felt insulted. 'All these stupid little tests! "Who's the Prime Minister?" "What day is it?" What do these people think I am – stupid?' (The truth is, at the time I was glad it was Mum doing the test, not me. I would have failed on the maths alone.)

Even so, I often wonder if I took the wrong path over the memory medication. There can be side effects – nausea, diarrhoea, insomnia, fainting – though they are expected to wear off. (I could be sure that if there were side effects Mum would get them all.) And at the time I was looking after Mum the positive effects on memory were expected to be temporary – about six months.

But had our GP been able to prescribe the memory medication I would have jumped at it too. It may even have helped with the depression. It was the process of acquiring the medication that would have been so difficult for us.

Other medication

For insomnia

Benzodiazepines are sometimes prescribed for short-term use. I didn't use any sleep medication for Mum; for people with dementia sleep medication can sometimes have the reverse effect. It can make them *race*. The guidelines for a person with dementia getting a good night's sleep are the same as for all of us – going to bed with not too many worries on the mind, a comfortable bed, maybe a heat pack to cuddle in the winter or a fan in the summer heatwaves.

---

[1] C. Bryden, *Dancing with Dementia: My Story of Living Positively with Dementia*, Jessica Kingsley Publishers, London, 2005, p. 29.

Psychosis and delusions

Antipsychotics may be recommended, usually Risperdal, Zyprexa, Seroquel.

Anxiety

They say buspirone is good anti-anxiety medication for people who are very nervous but do not have delusions, but, again, it can cause over-stimulation.

Depression

Antidepressants may be prescribed for depression.

- **Try to find a diary or calendar with BIG print and a clock or clocks with obvious symbols.**
- **Some people sew on Velcro fasteners to enable independent dressing, and buy shoes with Velcro straps or slip-on shoes.**

Where to seek help

You can contact **your GP, the local council and the local hospital.** The hospital will most likely have an Aged Care Assessment Team (ACAT) or will at least know where to access services. ACAT provide assessment, medical treatment (including assessment for 'memory' and other medication), carer's support, respite care and physical care. When we needed hand rails and a hand-held shower recess for the bathroom I accessed the Home Modification and Maintenance Service who worked in concert with an OT from ACAT. The local hospital may also run carer's groups and other support networks for carers.

The **Home Modification and Maintenance Service** (formerly the Home Handyman Service) will do jobs in the home for pensioners at subsidised rates.

The **Aids and Equipment Program** (formerly the Program of Appliances for Disabled People or PADP) – usually available through the local hospital. PADP will supply such equipment as wheelchairs, walking frames, hoists, continence aids. For most people there is an annual joining fee of $100 which will cover most costs.

Community Options – I used Community Options for the day centre and for in-house respite. (Lisa and then Susan.) They also ran a carers' support group, which met once a month.

Community Transport for outings, shopping expeditions and transport to and from some medical appointments. <http://www. cto.org.au/>.

Local **community centres** also provide social and support groups for senior citizens and their carers.

Chapter 2
Symptoms of dementia

Delusions

Dementia saps memory, but it can also cause anxiety, depression, agitation and delusions. A delusion is a fiction or fabrication that the person having the experience believes in implicitly. The person having the delusion believes the fiction is reality no matter what contradictory evidence there is and no matter what you say and do about it.

Some delusions initially appear to be happy things, for example, thinking that the Queen is coming for lunch. But if you really thought the Queen was coming for lunch it would be a source of angst. How would you cope? The house would have to be *spotless*. Who would accompany her? What would you serve for lunch? Would you pass muster? It's not such a happy thing after all.

When I started reading about the symptoms of dementia I rather optimistically thought that Mum was too logical to get delusions. All I would have to do would be to explain things to her and she would understand, I thought. I might have to explain a few times, I thought, but in the end she would understand. Then it hit. An outraged, decrepit old lady still recovering from a broken pelvis, seeing odd things in the house and wanting to 'go home' day and night. And so it really was not long before I found myself navigating around delusions.

The GP put her on the antipsychotic Zyprexa, which calmed her down a bit, but only a bit. I had to find other ways to cope with it.

Getting out of the house worked miracles. One day Mum was really going off. My sister took us out to the local nursery. It was a day of rare beautiful rain too. We wandered about, had coffee, got soaking wet looking at shrubs and seedlings. It was a good day. And back home Mum spent the afternoon drying wet clothes on our little oil heater. The delusion was shelved.

Getting Mum out of the house changed her thinking, took the panic away. When she wanted to go home and threatened to start walking, I would put her in the wheelchair and take her down to the supermarket. The checkout operators in the supermarket always talked to Mum. (They were factored into our support network. 'Where's your companion?' the deli lady would ask if I was on my own.) That usually helped Mum's thinking to change direction or at least it staved off the delusion for a while. Maybe once out she could see herself how difficult getting 'back to the other place' really would be just now, and she would change her mind. Then we'd go home and make dinner. That also helped.

When going home hit at night I would try putting it off. 'Think about it in the morning, Mum,' though it wasn't long before she was turning it back onto me. 'That's what you say about everything!' (She remembered that we had not gone home.)

'Well, there's nothing we can do tonight,' I would say. 'It's too cold/late/dark.'

'It certainly is cold.'

Where do delusions come from? With Mum they came hot on the heels of illness, unhappiness or a situation not understood. There is fear attached to delusions, fear of things left undone and fear of abandonment.

Insecurity, boredom and loneliness set them off. Even a television program would set off morbid thoughts in Mum if it was a bit slow. Too much change set them off, too many comings and goings of people she fancied might stay a while. But sometimes delusions seemed to appear just because. Something *clicked* and she was gone. A couple of hours later something clicked again and she was back.

There was a thread of logic to them, some connection with something else that had happened in real life. When she wanted to go home Mum often alternated between Campsie and Lakemba where she had lived as a child with her mother and sister. Another delusional haunt was Katoomba in the Blue Mountains, which my parents had both loved as a holiday destination. She would sometimes wake in the morning thinking that we were stuck in Katoomba and in need of getting home.

Overwhelmingly, however, Mum wanted to be back on our old farm at Wapengo in the Bega district, which she had owned and worked slavishly alongside my father. (My parents had been dairy farmers, first in Queensland and then in the Bega district, New South Wales.) The farm was sold in the 1970s, but logic had become subject to change now. After all, if Mum couldn't remember that her husband and son had died, where would she expect them to be? Home, of course. Home and needing dinner. There is logic to that.

I found that there was no right or wrong way to approach delusions, except that the calmer I was about them, the more *believing* I was, the quicker they went away and the less trauma there was along the way.

Some people go along with every bit of the delusion, no matter how elaborate it is. Others advocate the application of pure logic. They get out the death certificates of dead relatives: 'See, Mum? Grandma died in 1968. So you don't have to worry about getting home to Grandma. She isn't here any more.'

Logic never worked with Mum and only made her feel patronised, alienated.

I did a certain amount of lying or pretending, but only a certain amount. More often I just acted as if there was no problem at all and waited for it to go away, which is probably the same thing anyway.

If the person *is* convinced that the Queen is coming for lunch next week you could always try writing to the Palace including, of course, an explanatory note. A lady-in-waiting would certainly respond saying Her Majesty appreciates the support but unfortunately does not expect to be back in Australia this year. And then you would have a bona fide letter from the Palace to produce, no doubt regularly, to show there is no need to worry about having to make lunch for the Queen just now.

I used to find delusions pretty frightening. But delusions came and they went again. They could be fierce and elaborate, depending on her level of happiness and security and on her physical state. When she was sick and on antibiotics you could be sure that delusions would be zooming around outside our house like starved vampires seeking an open window. Still, they came and went.

> Trying to set straight the person having the delusion can really put a good wedge between the two of you, and it won't make any difference to the delusion. In the long run the delusion will still be there. A delusion can be overwhelming, the thing that will never leave, the thing that has you by the throat. Any passing exorcist would think he had come to the right place! But I found that delusions always left. And the calmer and quieter I approached them the quicker they left. One afternoon I looked at Mum afterwards and thought you would never know they had been here. The fog had dispersed yet again.

Memory and delusions

Mum was the only one left from her generation. Her mother died when I was a child. My father died in the late 1980s. Her sister and brother-in-law, my father's sister and brother-in-law, they were all gone. Mum could not remember. The stanchions that held memory in order were eroding.

'Is that you, Possy?' she called out practically every morning. (Her sister.)

'It's *me*!' I called back.

My brother Neil died in our own house. He keeled over from a cardiac arrest right in front of Mum. She could not remember.

My brother was one of the special thinkers. He had been diagnosed with schizophrenia when he was eighteen. We don't think he had schizophrenia, but that does not matter now. For all those years Mum had looked after him. Now she could not remember.

'Neil died,' we used to say when she puzzled over where he was and schemed over how to find him. It wasn't long, however, before we were saying as little as possible about Neil. It was not logical to her. If your son had died you think you would remember.

Often when things didn't make sense Mum came to her own conclusions and the conclusions became new delusions. Neil had not died – don't be so stupid! – but had simply left us. All we would have to do was track him down and lure him back, she thought. So it wasn't long before I was saying as little as possible about Neil.

Sometimes, however, she did remember.

'Did Uncle Harry die?'

'Yes, Mum.'

'Poor Poss! She must miss him terribly.'

So Uncle Harry was gone, but not Auntie Poss.

When it came to my father she decided he was off having an affair with a younger woman.

'How old would he have been now?' I would leap in. 'Can you seriously see him chasing after some woman? He wouldn't have even thought about it!'

'Well, where do you think he is?'

'He had cancer, Mum. You looked after him until he died. That was in the house in the inner city.'

'Yes, I know he had cancer, but ...'

Of course it did not sink in and sometimes caused awful rows, but it was the best I could think of. Sometimes she would recount something that one of the children had said after my father's funeral, but it did not stick. It was as if she couldn't afford for it to stick. To her they were just missing. Often she made up her mind that they simply didn't want to see her. They couldn't be bothered. And then I was leaping in again with distractions and explanations that could only ever offer short-term comfort. But short-term comfort is better than no comfort at all.

The Grandma delusion

When I was going through Mum's possessions I found some of the endless lists. There were the expected Christmas and birthday lists, and many of them. She had written them over and over, trying to remember who went where. Many were drawn up in what we would have called Mum's pre-dementia days, but I found that Grandma had been factored into them even then.

In fact, Grandma would feature prominently throughout those last three years. It was as if our regal grandmother had ventured back from the grave to keep order in the mayhem.

Mum would ask sometimes how I felt about the old lady coming to live with us. I said anybody could come and live with us.

But I remember one particularly sad Grandma-night early on. It had started about half past eleven in the night with Mum wanting to know where my father was. She was in her room, ready for bed. So I turned the lights out and went to bed myself, but it wasn't long before I heard her shuffling out. She went to the room in the middle of the house and called in whispers: 'Mother. Mother, can I come in? Are you alright? You don't look very comfortable.'

When I went to her she told me in a hushed voice that Grandma was sleeping on our verandah.

'Do you think she's warm enough?'

It was a very sad thing. 'Mum, it's one o'clock!'

'The mosquitoes are still up!' she defeated me. 'She has such fair skin.'

Then she was in and out getting pillows for a child she said was sleeping on the dining room table. She was making a barrier of pillows to stop him from falling off.

The next night she was waving to a child at the end of the hall. I saw her do it. A little boy, she said. (That was a happy episode for her.) She said the boy waved back. He was 'a nice little boy'.

That was when the GP suggested an antipsychotic, Zyprexa. After Zyprexa the nights were quieter. The little boy napping on the dining room table was gone at least.

As time went on Mum's increased frailty calmed the situation too. She could no longer physically roam the house to see if Grandma would like a cup of tea or to say goodnight to my father. She used me instead. 'Go and see if your father's alright, will you?'

At night-time she often wanted to know had I set dinner aside for Grandma. 'I don't know when she'll be in. Have you put her dinner in the oven?' I just said I had. What else can you say? The dead relatives were factored into our framework.

There was another time when Grandma was everywhere again. It took me a while to work out why. ANZAC Day was approaching. It was the power of association. ANZAC Day was something Grandma observed with fervour. Her brother had been killed in France and every year she had taken Mum and Auntie Poss in for the Dawn Service when they were little girls.

There were a lot of war documentaries and commentaries on the television as ANZAC Day neared and we were planning to go into town for the March. 'Mother made sure we took flowers to the Cenotaph on ANZAC Day in the colour of Uncle Will's regiment – purple and gold – and we all wore purple and gold ribbons,' she said. 'At school teachers made little flags with "Lest We Forget" and forgetmenots on for us kids who doled out cherished pennies for them and wore them on the day. School children ran stalls stocked with cut flowers and things to raise money for the returned soldiers.' She didn't seem to expect Grandma to turn up for the March though. She didn't ask about her coming with us. Maybe she thought Grandma would be too frail.

Sometimes I would make light of the spectres, though it was a risky business.

One night she was starting to fret. Have you seen Mother? Did you put dinner away for Mother? Have the visitors gone?

'We don't have any visitors, Mum,' I said.

'Oh, I'm glad they're gone.'

We were tucked up safe inside. 'We're all locked up for the night. I've locked the back door.'

'He might be cold out there.'

'Who?'

'Fa Fa.' Her grandfather.

'*Fa Fa!* Is there anybody else out there?' I said. 'What about the little girl from your primary school who got struck by lightning in the thunderstorm?'

'Parci Rhoban! At least I make you laugh!' she said, laughing herself.

With delusions I worked out the hard way that talking/discussing/ arguing was pointless. You have to keep it contained and stick to yes and no answers. That is not always a simple thing when you are confronted with direct questions.

Another day Mum thought she had been given money by somebody, 'The Matron', for buying eggs and something else from the supermarket but she could not remember what the something else was.

'Do you know how much money that woman gave me?'

'I don't think any woman gave you money, Mum.'

'I have to go and buy her eggs. Maybe I'll do it tomorrow when I can find out exactly what she wants.'

'She can buy her own eggs like I did for us today!'

Then she decided to go home. She thought home was in Fifth Avenue, Campsie, where she had lived as a child. She wanted to take a taxi back to Campsie.

'Where will you go from there? There are no motels in Campsie, Mother.'

She was exasperated with me. 'We'll take it from there.'

The egg-buying and going home had been going on since half past three. I said it was only a nightmare.

'If anybody comes looking for eggs,' I said, 'they can have some of our eggs. We'll share.'

'But the lady gave me money!'

'It was me who gave you the money, Mum. I put the money in your purse.'

'How much?'

'Thirty-five dollars.'

'God, they're expensive eggs!'

Then it was me who was exasperated. She had always defeated you with words. 'It was me who put the money in your purse – for your own sake. That's your own stash.'

She counted out the money. 'If I go home tonight what about the morning? We have to go and talk to the Matron who runs this place.'

'I don't know what you're talking about, Mum!'

'Oh! *Think*! Maybe *you* could go.'

'Where?' I said, thinking she meant the supermarket to buy the eggs. We had eggs already. We would share.

'Campsie.'

'I've never been to Campsie.'

'Oh, that doesn't matter,' she said in a comforting tone. 'You'd soon get used to it.'

'It will go away soon,' I whispered to the floorboards.

'Are you sure you don't want to come with me?'

'Where to?'

'Back to the other place! We can take a taxi.' She counted her money out again. 'And early in the morning we can talk to the lady.' Pause. 'Well? What are you going to do?'

'Nothing! I'm going to make us some dinner.'

'Alright. I'll wait until you've made dinner and then I'll go home. If I'm going to eat here I have to eat pretty close to straight away.'

At five o'clock she asked about her dinner. 'Is my dinner getting cooked?' she said with deliberate politeness.

'Yes. So is mine!'

'I know, my darling, but you may have to eat alone.'

There was another pause.

'If I don't have dinner soon I'll be in the dark.'

What did she really think? Was the tide that swept over her so strong and so awful that she had to go with it even though it didn't make *any* sense? She could not help it.

'I suppose I could always go tomorrow,' she said with a sigh. 'It's not as if they really need me.'

She was taking off her shoes. It was over.

Again, acceptance. Acceptance and lateral thinking. Acceptance is the only way. You go with the flow and it will eventually run dry.

The going home delusion

By November of that first year Mum was *really* going home. She had started 'phoning home'. She would wheedle our number out of me and then sit by the phone and dial the number. Of course she would get an engaged signal. 'At least we know somebody is there.'

She wanted somebody to help her move 'to the other place' and packed up the photos of the kids in readiness for leaving. She wrapped them in newspaper and put them in her suitcase. Even that seemed absurd, the precious things along with ruined stockings and other minor things stowed away in the massive suitcase going nowhere.

I found the online Eldercare Forum and sent them an SOS. Mum wants to go home all the time! What should I do? I did not understand their quiet responses to my frantic questions at the time. I understand them now. Basically the answer was you just have to wear it.

They were right. Going home took precedence over all other delusions and routinely I had to remind myself about how vile it would be to not know where you lived.

By August 2003 Mum was seeking out 'the proprietor' of *our* house to get him or her – the gender alternated – to make up our bill. She was terrified of running up a debt and wanted to pay off the owner so we could leave and go home unimpeded.

I wrote a letter. I was going to pretend the letter was from the spectral proprietor. In the letter I asked would she stay put. 'At present our own situation is in a state of flux and you would be doing me the greatest kindness if you would stay on until further notice,' I wrote on behalf of the phantom landlord. But I had doubts about lying to Mum like that.

So did my sister. 'Once you start doing such things you can't go back,' my sister said. 'Isn't it better to try and keep her in the here and now for as long as we can?' So I didn't deliver the letter and the thing is it probably wouldn't have helped much anyway. It might have helped for the moment, but it would not have been long before Mum would have been trying to track down 'this landlord person' to get the lowdown.

Some mornings she would look at objects in the house and identify them as hers with some surprise or relief: 'That's mine!' she would say, pointing out a lamp or the little porcelain jar she kept in the bathroom. 'That's mine too!'

'Of course it is!'

One morning we were having breakfast at the kitchen table with my niece and nephew when Mum began fussing about our suitcases, which she maintained were 'in the other place'. I could see where this was leading. How could we pack up and 'go home' if our suitcases were missing? The kids were there. We were having a leisurely big breakfast so it was easy. I said: 'Everything in this house is ours, Mum. Nothing's lost. Nothing's missing. Everything is here with us,' and quickly changed the subject to one of the young people.

Another time we went down to the shops with my sister and two of her boys who were going to get a hair cut. I wheeled her in view of Nick who was being shorn and she stopped and thought about the boy. She sat still for a moment and watched Nick talking footy with the barber. It relaxed its grip. All the tension in her face fell away and it was gone again.

One night our letter box was decapitated by a late night malcontent. In the morning Mum was bursting to go home so I wheeled her out the front so she could watch my sister hammer the letter box back into shape again.

Some episodes were less traumatising than others. One late afternoon she was drifting off into her own thoughts. 'I suppose if we tried to ring Brian (my father) to come and get us he'd be in the cow yard.' There was logic in that – he would not be able to come and get us if he was in the dairy!

Other times the going home delusions became elaborate nightmares that descended in the waking hours. I remember one time Mum gave me directions for getting home to the farm. (Perhaps she was feeling unable to go herself.) 'You walk down the road,' she instructed me, 'until you come to a fence that you have to climb over and hope the bull isn't there or that there are lots of cows to dilute his interest. Then you keep going north.' That is thinking that is well and truly entrenched. Nothing you can say will infiltrate it. No amount of reason will affect it. Again, all you can do is accept.

Another time we had returned home after a Community Transport outing and she felt stuck inside the house. She had cabin fever. A cold front was creeping up from the south with snow in Tasmania and Victoria. I thought that would be enough to keep her inside. In the afternoon she watched an episode of *Midsomer Murders* all the way through, tucked beside the heater, but the brilliant idea for what to do next was lacking and then it was on. 'I've got to get home tonight!'

So I took her down the street. She would not wrap up on good days least of all when she had been snared by a delusion. We needed things from the supermarket anyway. But another shopper asked her about the wheelchair. 'How long have you been in a wheelchair?' Of course Mum couldn't answer such a question and the last thing she needed reminding of was her own frailty. The delusion flared up again.

We went through the checkout and I turned the wheelchair into our street.

'Where are we going now?'

'Home,' I said.

'Oh! Home!' she humphed. What I called home and what Mum called home could be two or more separate things.

She ate her dinner happily that night, tucked up beside the heater again. (She normally wouldn't eat anything when she had delusions.) It went on most of the night, though I just calmly ignored it. Mum was waiting for my brother-in-law to get home from work so that he could 'come and get us'. She wrapped things up in plastic bags in readiness. And I just ignored it. It was getting late. I put on her electric blanket in readiness for sleep.

Finally *Glass House* came on the TV. The cast were doing a Costello versus Howard skit. There was something about Peter Costello putting up a ransom for John Howard's head on a platter. 'No price is too high,' was the doctored Costello's response and Mum laughed outright. Laughter released the safety valve. She was fine again and went into bed.

'Sweet dreams,' she said as I turned her light out.

'Yeah, you too, Mum.'

The baby delusion

My mother was not the first person with dementia to experience the baby delusion and I doubt she will have been the last.

The baby delusion was also set off by association. It was August 2004. We needed to get a birthday gift for my sister. So Lisa, the respite worker, gave us a lift to the shopping centre so that we could buy a gift.

Lisa and I were talking about an adoption story that had been on television. Also, there was a baby in his stroller in the lift and that was, I think, how the idea crept into Mum's head. That afternoon she told me secretively, somewhat sheepishly, that she was having a baby herself. It was hard to keep the news quiet, she said.

What do you do? I decided to play it down, to just ignore it. I figured if I went along with it I would not be doing her any favours and it would be hard for her to get out of it again. I figured I would just try and contain it. I knew it would upset others. People are squeamish. Also, it is the extreme abnormality of the condition of dementia smacking you in the face.

So I just ignored it. Now I think what I should have done was treat the thing with absolute pragmatism and gone and bought her a test.

I can see myself now getting out the test. 'You're not, Mum. Never mind. Probably just as well. We have enough to do, don't we, without a baby to take care of.'

She certainly would have protested. 'Have you read the instructions properly?'

'Yes, we've read the instructions. We'll do it again tomorrow if you need to be sure.' And then I could have put it aside and taken her out or found her occupations sufficiently interesting to take her mind off it.

- **Try and contain anger and irritation. There is no such thing as compromise anymore. Your upset will only increase her upset.**
- **Trying to infiltrate the delusion and dispel it with logic almost certainly will never work.**
- **What does it matter if you don't understand it?**
- **Try to remember that it's the illness talking.**

Agitation

Severe agitation is said to be a main reason that families eventually seek a nursing home for the person they care for.

Symptoms of agitation can include:

- irritability, frustration, rage, lashing out with words or blows
- over the top reactions
- constant demands for attention and reassurance

- repetitive questions or telephone calls
- stubborn refusal to respond to reasonable requests, for example, showering or going out
- constant pacing, searching, rummaging, secreting things away.

Mary Summer Rain, author of *Love Never Sleeps*, outlined many agitation-specific problems that she and her fellow carer faced when they undertook the role of caring for the friend's mother.[2] For example, Mum expected to be able to share her meals with her dog and would either throw violent tantrums or refuse to eat herself if the carers would not let her share with the dog. She would stow food away in her clothes and everywhere else.

What would you do? Maybe you could try taking a plate to the table, a human plate, not the dog's bowl. 'Okay, Mum. This is the dog's plate. If you take the piece of fish out of your pocket and put it on her plate we can put it in the fridge and save it for the dog.' And at the end of the day you help her take the plate from the fridge and scoop the food into the dog's bowl.

It may not have *worked*. There would still have been the endless questions of 'have you fed the dog?' You might have to take her to the fridge ten times to show her that the food was still there. It may not have solved the problem of Mum overfeeding the dog while underfeeding herself, but it may well have helped in maintaining a calm atmosphere around meal times, an atmosphere that, ideally, would flow over into other aspects of daily life.

Sudden illnesses such as bladder infections or colds or toxic reactions to medication can cause increased confusion and agitation.

A noisy and poorly lit environment can increase the unhappiness of a dependent person. A cheerful environment goes a long way to creating calm and peace.

Hospitalisations and other dramatic changes to normal living

---

[2] M.S. Rain, *Love Never Sleeps: Living at Home with Alzheimer's*, Hampton Roads Publishing Company Inc., Charlottesville, VA, 2002, p. 83 and p. 118.

can cause agitation.

Feeling overwhelmed by numbers of people or by abstract debate can cause upset.

Feeling cold can cause upset.

But so can disappointment, loneliness and fear. Being left alone for long periods is likely to cause major upset to the person with dementia. My mother could not be safely left alone for very long at all.

She was not always tolerant anymore either. One night we went over with Carly (niece) to watch *Pirates of the Caribbean* with my sister's boys. It was a funny and lively film, but it was very long and Mum thought it was rubbish.

She was going home, she said. She wanted to go home. She had work to do! 'Can't you imagine the rest?' she finally said, sulking. That was not Mum at all. The old Mum would have done anything for the young people.

- **I found that the more occupied Mum was, the more relaxed she remained.**
- **Believing or accepting her take on things went a long way towards calming combativeness.**
- **Ask if the person would like help. Or compromise. Don't necessarily just take over. You may be going against their wishes and then you'll be wondering why all the storms! In other words, don't assume the person has abandoned all hope of making decisions for themselves.**

Coping with change

Change isn't good for people with dementia. Even characters from new television programs may not be absorbed. Inspectors Frost (*A Touch of Frost*) and Barnaby (*Midsomer Murders*) were like old friends to my mother. But Inspector Foyle from *Foyle's War* did not pass inspection. *Foyle's War* was new and unknown so she would not watch it. There were no established ties, I expect.

In the middle of 2004 Carly, the same niece, decided to stay with us for a while.

'Carly is going to live with us for a while,' I told Mum.

'If it's alright, Gran.'

'Of course, darling!'

When Carly moved in there was a lot of noise and activity. We watched late night movies together.

'Listen to her, Mum!'

'What's she singing?'

'"I like Aeroplane Jelly"!'

'She's a gorgeous girl. Full of life!'

Mum loved having Carly, though the change made her confused and her miseries started growing in strength. All the comings and goings were a bit much for her. 'Is Carly in for dinner?' 'Is Carly coming home?' 'Do you think Carly is alright?'

Another dramatic change was meeting Susan, the adult daughter of my grandmother's ex-husband. It's a bit of a story. When Mum was a baby her father died from the Spanish flu. Grandma remarried a younger man called Teddy, but the marriage didn't work. After the divorce Teddy and Grandma had remained friends. She was even friends with Teddy's new wife and maintained contact with them all including their own daughter, Susan. To Susan our grandmother had been 'Auntie Jessie' and a cloak of secrecy had been drawn over the rest of it. We had heard of Susan but she didn't know we existed and had only recently discovered that her father had been married before, married with two little stepchildren, in fact – Mum and Auntie Poss. She had gone to some efforts to track Mum down.

In May Susan came to our place and met the three of us, regretting, of course, that Mum had become 'so fragile' before they finally met up as 'stepsisters'. Mum understood who Susan was and was glad to meet her.

In July it was our turn to repay the call. Mum coped well enough. She looked at a photo of Teddy and his brothers and said the brother Dan had red hair. Susan swung around: 'Yes, that's right! Dan had red hair!'

After the visit, however, Mum claimed Susan's husband Ron as her long-gone stepfather and could not be talked out of that.

'It must have been interesting for Teddy to see us grown up.'

'That was Ron, Mum, Susan's husband.'

'I'm talking about Teddy. Teddy was very fit. He did shift work on the railways. Of course, Mother was never home. He took us to the beach. That was brave of him, two little girls in tow who weren't even his.'

Teddy became another spectre in our lives, but it did not really matter too much except that he had been so strongly connected with my grandmother who was already a spectre in our lives.

To the end Mum knew who Susan was. The last time she was in hospital was just after Christmas. I took her a gift from Susan. Susan had made her a chiffon shawl.

'She dyed the material herself, Mum.'

'That was very nice of Susan,' she said. 'Susan is very creative.'

Yes, she knew who Susan was.

Fear and insecurities

Anxious people worry about losing things. They worry about being late for appointments. They worry that loved ones may have met with foul play. They worry about being abandoned. They worry about worrying.

It was extremely important for Mum to see that I was alright. And that I was alright with her.

Early on I went out to a concert. The Rolling Stones had come to town and off I went with my other brother, Paul, and two of his adult children, Carly and Josh. Ra, my sister, sat with Mum that night, but could not get her into bed. We were home late and Mum had to stay up and wait. She had to be sure that I was still in one piece before she could relax enough to go to bed herself.

The insecurities took a lot of reassurance.

'Where are the keys? I can't find the keys! Oh, you have them. Are they the keys to this house?'

'Yes, Mum.'

'Do you have keys to the other house?'

'These are the only keys we have.'

'How puzzling!'

She was also becoming a bit paranoid. She decided one day that somebody had been at her bankbook. She named the person of her suspicions. That person, a troubled personality, had phoned to talk to her and Mum had glued the two things together.

'It was me, Mum,' I tried to explain. 'I had to take your bankbook so I could go and take out your pension.' She wasn't listening. 'That woman! She's so officious. She just said: "Give me your bankbook. I'm going to take out your pension!" I don't mind helping, of course. I just object to her attitude.'

That was startling. Mum would say to me that I looked after her 'very well'.

'It was me, Mum!' I said. 'I had to take out the money.'

'Oh, it was that woman! She's been here all afternoon.'

That was me too.

Some days were worse than others, of course. Mum was restless one night. We needed things from the supermarket anyway, so I wheeled her down. She was frightened of the dark, even though I was there pushing her and the moon was full in the sky. The street was too dark for her. Every shadow hid things unknown.

It was certainly better to go to the shops in the daylight. And she drew the attention of little children in the supermarket. 'I am about their level!' she would laugh, and we made jokes about not asking for sweets when we went through the checkout.

We passed a couple with a toddler one day.

'What did that little girl say?'

'"Lady in a pram"!'

She laughed. 'The little pet!'

Another day we went to Parramatta with Carly and another

niece, Liz. Carly had a job interview and the rest of us went to Westfields to fill in the time. In Westfields I felt that the walls were moving in on me, but Mum loved it. She enjoyed herself. We had coffee, then collected Carly and drove home to Liz's flat. It was a splendid place looking over a playing field with trees everywhere. I don't remember which level we were on, but Mum was terrified. She thought I would fall off their balcony. 'Come away! Come away from the balcony! Come away!'

One birthday my brother, Paul, gave her money. 'I'm afraid my present is very boring, Mum,' Paul said, and then he handed her a card with a hundred dollar bill inside.

'Boring?' At the time she shone like the Lighthouse of Alexandria. But she was very protective of that money.

'Will you get it changed into two fifties?'

We went down to the shops and had it changed.

'Will you look after them? Maybe you'd better keep one safe for me. Perhaps you should keep them both. Maybe I should keep one. No, they are probably both safer with you.' An hour later came the first of many enquiries. 'Do you still have the money?'

Of course there were some things that would have upset anybody. There was an injury to Mum's arm one day en route to the day centre. It seems the wheelchair wasn't properly secured and when the bus went round a corner it leapt. Mum had put her arm out to stop it from falling and it ripped off a great patch of skin on her arm. At the centre they had wrapped it up, but it was a bad one. Blood had soaked through the bandages and I hurt her just getting her cardigan off when she came home in the afternoon.

The following morning we soaked it in a dish of warm water but the bandage they had put on stuck like cement. I gave her asprin to try and take her mind off it. We finally prized the bandage off using vaseline. The wound was bleeding and pretty massive so I asked the doctor to pay a visit. He said to cover it again and leave it for 48 hours. So I covered it and left it.

Forty-eight hours later it was my turn to get the bandages off after soaking. We had put medicated gauze under ouchless bandages and this time the gauze was stuck like super glue. I gave her asprin again and she was uncomplaining though it stuck and stuck to the old skin. And when the gauze finally came off blood spurted everywhere again. So I left it uncovered in the hope that it would form a blood-scab. I knew the new medical advice was to bandage a wound, but getting the bandages off was causing her suffering so I left it. In the night she was fussing about it, of course.

'I want it covered. It needs to be covered!'

'But if I cover it again, Mum, the bandages will stick again and it'll hurt like blue blazes getting it all off again.'

'Better that than going to bed with an arm dripping puss!' (There was a great bloody sponge of bruise about it, which she took for infection.)

'It's not infection, Mum. The blood is scabbing over, which is good. It'll heal now.' (I hoped.) 'All the red is just bruise.'

The blood-scab made people gasp, but I still think bandaging and unwrapping would have been torture for her. Within a month much of the scab had fallen away. It left a reminding scar of bright pink flesh, but at least there was no infection.

There can also be anxiety caused by the thoughtlessness of others. One evening some kids threw bungers from their car as they sped passed our house and Mum nearly went through the roof. 'What is it? What is it?'

I rushed over to her. 'It's just kids!'

'Are you sure? It sounded like the roof was falling in!'

'It's just kids throwing bungers.'

'That was so loud.'

Yes, it was. I could have throttled them.

There may be fear over change and feelings of incapacity. In September 2005 Paul and Di, my brother and sister-in-law, went on a six-week holiday overseas and Mum fretted and fretted over that. For a while I wished I hadn't told her they were going.

She was very stressed. She couldn't remember who was going. If it was Ra and Col, who would look after the boys? 'We don't have instructions for the children!' she said often and was very anxious – school lunches, school uniforms. 'Ra hasn't left instructions!'

'Ra and Col aren't going anywhere,' I told her.

'Are you sure?'

'Absolutely. Paul and Di have gone overseas. And their kids are old enough to look after themselves, aren't they?'

'Yes, *they* are.'

'It's alright. Ra and Col aren't going anywhere.'

'Oh! What a relief! Thank goodness for that.' She calmed down for a while.

At that time the weather was bad so we spent the next day working in the house. I decided to rearrange the study. I moved the furniture while Mum sat at the table in the wheelchair. I brought her dampened tea towels and she cleaned off the books. And then she handed them back for re-shelving.

I thought we had done good work, but that night she was really getting the heebie jeebies about who was where, who had gone overseas, who was lost, not lost. It was late enough for bed, but she was wretched and couldn't sleep. So I went in and read to her. I read until she fell asleep. (When I crept out a board creaked, but it didn't wake her.) And I told myself, remember this. You remember this. If she was in care and got the heebies she would be told to stay in bed, gone crook on, maybe restrained. You remember this, I said. I'm so lucky. It was just so lucky.

The next morning Ra wrote big letters on an envelope and sticky taped it on Mum's work table: 'Only Paul and Di have gone to London. Nobody else.' We kept that on her work table until they came home.

Wandering and pacing

Christine Bryden, who has fronto-temporal dementia, wrote that she will often 'get very distracted and agitated, for no apparent reason, but it seems to arise mainly from this undercurrent of lack of recall and possible forgetting of something important. So I pace around almost like a caged lion, or simply can't sit still, particularly in the evening... I find it difficult to settle at night, probably because it is hard to follow the story on TV, the adverts are noisy and disturbing, and even reading is tiring and difficult.'[3]

So wandering can be associated with gaps in the memory as well as delusions. And it is when people roam that they are unsafe. Some carers find themselves having to put away knives and other sharps, having to deadlock doors and take the knobs off the stove in the night.

Mum felt she had to do something, usually something to look after me or the missing family members. Of course I was always nearby so she did not have to go far. When she felt secure and knew that we were safe, the house was locked up, the heaters turned off, she was fine. She stopped roaming the house looking for deceased relatives after taking the antipsychotic Zyprexa. Also, as I have said, her immobility would have made roaming difficult. Not that it would have stopped her trying. Had I not been there she would have gone off, fallen and ended up in hospital yet again.

- **Unexpected changes or having to rush can cause fear and disorientation.**
- **Some people suffer from paranoia, for example, thinking somebody is stealing their money or possessions or lying to them.**
- **Exercise helps with general well-being. Try to get some gentle walking in every day.**
- **Pleasant activities, perhaps patting the dog or listening to music – nothing too melancholy – or playing simple card games, can all help promote calm.**
- **Keep things simple. Give her the easy jobs that you know she can do.**
- **Distract with a favoured DVD or a snack or with a favoured topic of conversation.**
- **Try not to put the person in a position where demands – including jokes and conversation – will be beyond them now.**

---

3 Bryden, *ibid,* p. 113.

Depression

People with depression can also have delusions, thinking that they are ill, that they have been abandoned by everyone, or have lost their money. Mum was often looking for her mother and other relatives, thinking she had to look after them now.

When depression was bad for Mum I found her jobs to do. She sorted the washing. She folded the towels and matched one sock to another. She dried clothes and tea towels on the little oil heater. I took the knives and forks in to her in the colander so she could dry them at her little work table in the lounge room. When I was making a white sauce to go with dinner she chopped the parsley. She sliced the capsicums and onions, grated the cheese. All those things are her jobs and she expected them to be her jobs.

But the fits of depression were much harder than delusions. To borrow one of Mum's own expressions, she went from being a happy and resilient person to somebody 'stewing in a broth of trouble'. I would get frustrated with it and then turn around and feel entirely sorry for her.

But it is easy for older people to suffer despair. There may be loneliness, of course. In our family everybody else her own age was gone. And Mum was once so active. She ran the house, tended her beloved garden, she looked after Neil. She had always done voluntary work. She always read and laughed and talked and fed people. She had always been the one to look after others. She had been *so* active. But now she was frail and the frailty came back as a rotten reminder of her prior life.

'I'm useless!'

'Just because the old legs don't go *at the moment* doesn't mean you're useless! You're still Grandma, aren't you?'

'Oh yes, I suppose, but …'

Then I would find her a job. Jobs were good. Sometimes I put on a load of washing just so that Mum could dry the things on the heater and have a feeling of occupation. She sometimes complained. 'All this washing!' And then she got stuck in drying it all on the heater.

In the sunlight I wheeled her and the green Sulo bin out into the front garden and we binned garden refuse. There was always something to do in the garden.

Inside I could wheel her to the kitchen where the portable CD player lived. We played favoured arias and the 'William Tell Overture' and 'Land of Hope and Glory' and 'Jupiter' from the *Planets Suite* quite loudly. 'You have to play it loud, Mother!' I'd say. There we did the washing up together. I washed and put the things on the table. She dried. I put away. 'What next?' she would say when that task was done.

I remember one afternoon we had a small adventure. We were coming back from the shops and Mum was depressed. But we found two very young boys out in the street playing. I parked Mum on our side of the street and went across to speak to them, but they didn't speak much *Human*.

'Where's your Mummy?' I asked the bigger one.

'Mummy!' he said back.

'Is Mummy at the shops?'

'Sopps!'

Nobody answered the door of the house they seemed to belong to. I went next door, herding them along with me. I bashed on the door. No answer. I bashed again on the door. No answer. What do you do? I could hardly take them home with me! And some people hoon down our street quite oblivious so I could hardly leave them there either. They were nice little kids. I wheeled Mum over, told the little one to 'stay with Grandma'.

'Gamma!' So Mum sat in the wheelchair and talked to the little one and he didn't take off.

I went and knocked on the first door again. Grandpa emerged. Hallelujah! They were alright, and our small adventure changed Mum's thinking, gave her something else to think on – she was always brilliant with children – and dispersed the black fog yet again.

Keeping busy

Keeping busy is a good antidote for depression. One night I started reading out loud. There was a blackout and I picked up Winston Graham's *Poldark* and started reading by candle light.

'Keep going,' Mum said. When the lights came back on we read the book properly. Nearly three chapters in and she was still listening. The characters were old friends, just as some actors become old friends. After that I read to her day and night.

Sometimes for birthday teas we would make a cake together. Mum sat at the table in the wheelchair and I gave her the cake mixture and the beaters so she could do the frosting.

When it was time for kerbside pick-up we collected a nephew or two and went scrounging. It made for interesting walks. Cars would be cruising the pick-up and we too would search for treasure.

Sometimes we would join the family when they went around to the park to play cricket. One dull weekend we went and played a game with Nick, the youngest nephew, and Col, brother-in-law. Nick had new cricket gear and wanted to try it out. So we went down to the school playground. We pushed the wheelchair right up onto the green and there Mum sat happily minding the dog. (To the end she talked cheerfully about our cricket match. 'Remember when we went to the school and the boy played cricket? We should do that again.')

In the splendid spring days I wheeled Mum about the neighbourhood and we gaped together at the batches of wisteria coming into bloom. Our wayward jasmine hung like a tarpaulin over the trees. The perfume overtook us as soon we went out the front door.

At home we sat on our front verandah and potted seedlings. There was always something to talk about.

'The petunias are budding up, Mother.'

'Are they those nice red ones?'

'They're the red ones.'

But it was difficult to stay occupied on hot or rainy days. Those times again I realised how much time we spent outside.

One day when the respite worker came I left her and Mum talking and went to the local haberdashery shop. I bought some beads, pink and blue, in the hope that Mum might string them – always looking for something to do. They weren't big enough. But in the night I dug them out and Mum began to string them. The pink ones were bigger. She strung them and there was a bracelet. The others were smaller and harder on the old eyes, though she had a go. I said we would make jewellery for Christmas gifts. The old eyes would not go the full distance and I finished off the job. But it was a good idea.

She could no longer knit either. She might work at something with enthusiasm for a couple of days and then toss the project aside. We tried to knit squares for a rug, but Mum kept undoing the knitting, saying it was no good. I thought it didn't matter whether the knitting was any good or not, but Mum did. She simply could not do it anymore.

For months, however, she was making picture books 'for the poor children', exercise books filled with pictures that she cut from magazines. That was a wonderful project and it kept her occupied for hours on rainy days. But one day she just set them aside and refused to go back to them.

In December we might make Christmas goodies. That last December we made shortbread and mince pies. I cut out the pastry for the pies. 'Little stars!' she laughed over the finished project. Some looked more like little octopuses to me, but no matter.

We decided together which Christmas and birthday gifts we would buy when we went on our sojourns to the shopping centre. That last Christmas there were extra chocolates to buy and wrap, gifts for Other Susan, the new respite worker, and the Community Transport drivers, 'The Bus Boys'. There was always somebody else to think about.

- Encouraging a person to try and stick at activities they can't do anymore only promotes frustration. Nobody needs to be reminded of what they can no longer do.
- Some activities may be very short term.
- Try and keep something up your sleeve in readiness for low moods, perhaps a favoured DVD.

Pet therapy

One day my niece, Liz, asked if I'd like another cat for my birthday. I forgot all about it until the next time Liz visited, looking pretty and excited. 'Happy birthday, Mems!' She handed over a miniscule tortoiseshell kitten, rescued by the local Cat Lady. Molly.

Molly was insufferable. She would hide behind doors and leap on me, purring of course, to shred my skin. So I went and bought her a companion, a fat healthy companion, all white except for ginger ears and a ginger tail, which looked like it had been glued on. Mum looked him over.

'I was thinking of calling him Eddie, Mother.'

'Charlie!' she said. 'Charlie's a good name for him.'

And when he had a toileting mishap she made allowances. 'He couldn't help it. We've got to expect some problems.'

Molly and Charlie became inseparable. There were aspects about them that Mum found very entertaining. She was frightened by the family's dog now when he was off the leash, frightened that he would knock her over. But the kittens were another matter. They would curl up on her bed with their paws around each other's necks. 'Will you look at this? Aren't they gorgeous? That's what was wrong with Molly!' she would say.

When one of my sister's cats took out a fatwa on the kittens Mum would offer words of comfort. 'Did she get you, love? Now you're alright!' The kittens were family.

Pets can be company, comfort and a talking point. There were other times when the kittens drove Mum crazy though. 'The noise of them! Always rampaging about! I know they can't help it, but really!' The kittens were naughty. They did a lot of rough-house and raced up and down the hall like ponies trying to outrun each other. It was those times when she would get fed up with them. 'Why can't they go outside?' So I would shut them in the back part of the house and they would rampage out there.

Other times they retreated under her bed. Of course when Mum was getting into bed herself the cats would let us know they were there.

'Grandma, you're purring!' I'd say, tucking her in.

'It isn't me! Would you mind removing them?'

The February storms frightened the daylights out of Molly. I remember one night making her a hidey-hole in the linen cupboard and she stayed there for a long time but a great crash of thunder brought her hurtling out and she relocated under Mum's bed.

'Poor Moll!' Mum said, then instantly changed direction. 'I wonder how the calves are getting on. But they don't seem to worry about such things. Do you know where Brian is?'

'No, Mum.'

'I hope he's not out in the rain.'

'Nobody is out in the rain,' I told her. 'Not even Charlie!' (Charlie is a Turkish Van. Turkish Vans are renowned for their special fondness for water. Charlie was quite likely to be out in the storm enjoying the spectacle.) And she laughed. Laughter released the safety valve again.

Chapter 3
Personal care

Working it all out

It took me too long to fathom how much help Mum needed now. I remember early on we took her down to the local arcade to get her hair cut. It took her two hours to get ready for that. I had made an appointment, but we were very late. I hadn't yet worked out that I had to just take over and say these slacks, that top, here are your shoes and stockings, okay, we'll brush your hair. Let's go.

We did get there and Mum did get her hair cut. She was very gracious about it.

'I'm lucky to have you,' she said that night. (I was lucky to have her.)

I was getting her last cup of tea for the night. 'You must be getting sick of this – having to make me tea and things. Thank you, darling. I'll be better soon.'

'Don't worry about it, Mother. You'll be better soon.'

I confess when I realised she needed help to dress I found it repugnant at first. It's a progression, I said to myself. You get used to these things, I told myself. And you certainly do.

One day she was calling me and I found her coming out of the bathroom with a towel around her. She was cold and wanted to get into my bed. She needed me. I helped her get into her warm gown and took her into the lounge room and warmed her in front of the heater.

It wasn't that long before I was helping her put her clothes on and doing everything else without a second thought. Some of it was another endurance test, but only because of repetition.

The only real problem was getting her in the shower. It's a common problem and many people call on respite workers to help with showering, but that only made Mum feel put upon.

Showering

The Home Modification and Maintenance Service installed a hand-held shower and safety railing in the bathroom. My sister-in-law, Di, is a physiotherapist and she gave us a shower chair. The shower chair is a great invention but is, of course, made of plastic and plastic can be cold to sit on. I would lay a hand towel or washer over it and heat them up with the shower nozzle *first* before getting Mum into the shower recess. When the weather was cold I warmed towels on the oil heater.

Still, getting Mum in the shower now became very difficult. She just hated it. She was afraid of falling, of course. She was most likely afraid of everything, but especially of falling though she had the shower chair to perch on and me to lean on. It was the getting in and out part that she was frightened of, though I held her up, of course.

Another problem was feeling the cold. The hand-held shower was good but did not give all-over warmth. I had to get her out of the shower and wrapped in towels pretty quickly otherwise she would be instantly cold.

Mum also objected to being told what to do. Instead of 'do you want to have a shower?' I would try: 'Oh, it's shower time! I'll run the water for you.' I used to be able to kid her into washing her hair herself: 'Here's the Pears shampoo that one of the kids gave you for Christmas. Put your hand out.'

I used to be able to get her singing in the shower. She'd sing 'Rule Britannia', laughing at herself – or me – but no longer. It was not long before she would just get stroppy and terribly offended. I had to try to not laugh at the things she bellowed at me.

Often I couldn't get her in the shower at all. Bathing then comes down to a wash.

Continence aids

The chemist and the supermarket stock Tenas and Depends, protective pull-up pants. These are not washable or recyclable.

PADP supply up to 80 pads a month, I believe, but they have a waiting list. PADP will also supply a commode, so if the person needs to get up in the night she won't have far to go.

Skin care

Older people are susceptible to thrush and other muck that gets into crevices, especially after a course of antibiotics. Antifungal creams are gentle, available from the chemist and they do the job.

Skin can often become dry, making it itchy and uncomfortable. A good moisturiser for hands and body after showering or before bed keeps skin supple and comfortable. A lavender skin lotion will smell good too. But you have to watch some perfumed lotions that can burn sensitive or old skin. It's best to test a small patch on the arm first before ladelling it on.

Frailty

When Mum came home from hospital in September 2002 her broken pelvis was the immediate medical problem.

The Home Modification and Maintenance Service, working in concert with the hospital OT, put up hand rails at the back door as well as in the shower. Mum was pretty good for the workers who came to the house. The physio took her for walks down the road on a frame and seemed to cope well enough when Mum hounded her for crutches. She had had crutches years earlier for her hip replacement that had gone poorly and she wanted crutches again now. Crutches would make everything better, she thought.

Nieces Liv and Carly had a rented house in the suburb next to us then and we went there for a birthday celebration. Getting Mum up the stairs leading to the house was a bit like negotiating the Mount Lofty Ranges, but we managed.

But Mum's increasing frailty became a challenge to me and a source of misery for her. We both had a difficult time adjusting to frailty. I remember one day when my sister took us to a local shopping centre and Mum sulked about getting in the complimentary wheelchair. 'I'll look like an old person!'

By September 2004, however, we needed the wheelchair for getting around inside the house as well as outside. The wheelchair took some getting used to but it made life so much easier. To exit the house we went out the back through the kitchen. We did not have ramps so she clambered out and I helped her down the back steps where she stood holding onto the rail while I brought the wheelchair down so she could get back in. 'I suppose you get some exercise that way, Mother!' To get her out the front to sit in the sun on the verandah I opened the front door and pushed her out, bump, bump. 'Sorry, Mother.' (Being pushed in a wheelchair requires a bit of trust.) And then out the front we could work on the pot plants or just watch others passing by.

When I had to nip off to the shops for milk or cat food I always made sure Mum knew where I was headed.

'I'm just going to the shops, Mother. I won't be long. Will you sit tight?'

'I'll sit right here till you get back.'

'Promise?'

'I promise!'

And mostly she did. Still I rushed. One morning I rushed passed Lonely Man (an uncommunicative local) who gave me his usual glare as I tore passed.

'I'm not going to bother with Lonely Man anymore, Mum,' I whinged when I came home. 'I try and give him a smile or a g'day …'

'Some people are just rude. Maybe that's why they call him Lonely Man.'

'It's me who calls him Lonely Man.'

'Why do you call him that?'

'Because I figured he'd be lonely!' She laughed.

But one night she gave me a ticking off for being too rough while helping her to bed.

'Thanks …'

'No worries, Blue,' I said, as usual. But she hadn't finished.

'… for nothing!' she added. 'You haul me around like a sack of potatoes!'

That was embarrassing. Normally she said 'sweet dreams' or 'you get to bed too'. But it was good she spoke up. I hadn't known I was being rough.

Falls

Falls and broken bones are debilitating. Often the person believes they have more capabilities than they really do and so falls are common. And you hear people say 'it was the last fall that did it.'

The essentials for people with poor mobility are sensible shoes, appropriate walking aids, including frames, and a 'Grandma-proof' living environment. In other words, making sure there are no obstructions, even phone cords and rugs, anything that can trip the person up.

The walking stick is preferred over the quad stick, which is heavy and easier to trip over.

Simple exercises

A gentle exercise program for elderly people includes walking, even if it is only a tour of the house twice a day on your arm.

For strengthening leg muscles try leg lifts and stand ups – standing from a seated position by pressing hands on knees and pushing up with thighs.

For the sake of circulation keep legs elevated if possible. Heel and toe exercises keep the ankles moving.

Arm raises. Lift arms forward and up above the head. Press back at the top to work upper back muscles.

Diagonal isometric bracing. With foot off floor press onto opposite knee. Fight the tension to strengthen stomach muscles. Hold for a couple of seconds. Relax. Repeat three to five times with each foot.

It sounds all well and good, but it isn't always possible to get the person to comply.

Bladder infections (UTIs)

Increased confusion and fever may indicate a urinary tract infection. People with infections are more prone to physical immobility, falls and increased confusion. My mother was often on antibiotics for UTIs. I learned to spot the symptoms so I could nip down to the doctor and get Mum antibiotics. (I kept a specimen jar in the bathroom in readiness.)

I remember one time a high fever came over Mum all of a sudden and she was in real misery. I rugged her up, gave her asprin to get the fever down and raced down to the doctor to get her Keflex.

Ulcers and bed sores

Immobility and poor circulation make people susceptible to *deep* infections. In February 2005 Mum was brewing an ulcer on her ankle, probably from hitting herself on the paddles of the wheelchair, the 'stirrups'.

The new theory is that a wound has better hope of repairing itself in a wet environment. So the treatment for ulcers is Duoderm patches. They are available from the chemist, but they are expensive and make the wound mushy. I put on a patch and then it became very obvious indeed.

And it was bad. 'Ulcers are rotten things,' I had heard right throughout my childhood. I had heard about the Changi POWs having their ulcers scraped out for them. 'Ulcers are just dreadful!' And now I knew for myself.

Keflex didn't help it. And her foot was turning a bit rotten looking. Her toes looked like red sausages. There was a poison mark going up the leg. My sister marked the redness with pen so we could track it and see if it was getting worse. I made some stupid throwaway line about amputation and then Mum was thinking she would lose her foot.

'You're not going to lose your foot, Mum! I was just mucking around. Honestly! I was just being stupid!'

'I'm not so sure.'

'Mum! I was just being stupid! It was just a stupid joke.'

Yes, what a stupid joke.

The doctor ordered an ultrasound, which showed that the bone was not affected. She didn't need hospital. Two courses of penicillin killed the infection. But, of course, there were delusions.

Finally that ulcer dried up and the delusions lifted and we were laughing again. I took her back to the doctor for a check-up. He said it looked good but to try and keep her legs elevated.

The next morning I set her up in front of *Little House on the Prairie* on TV, pulling up the wheelchair as a footstool.

'Is that comfortable?'

'Yes, it's comfortable, but now I can't see the television!' And she doubled over laughing again.

As time went on there were other ulcers, always on her ankles.

The old treatment for ulcers was five minutes in the sun every day. I wish I had thought of that simple remedy when I was looking after my mother. I'm sure it would have made all the difference. Five minutes in the sun every day.

- **Give adequate pain relief.**
- **Remember physical comfort as well as emotional security. Older people may feel the cold and may need a night light.**
- **Get a flu needle for you both.**
- **Watch out for UTIs and other infections.**
- **When showering is impossible make do with a wash – hands, face and toosh.**

Medications

The chemist put the daily medication in blister packs so I could dispense them easily – breakfast, lunch, dinner. (You take the empty packs back to the chemist for refilling.)

When the heart medication Vioox was banned I took the tablets out of her blister pack straight away. The chemist replaced Vioox with Celebrex and almost immediately Mum was feeling drab and nauseous. She would be lying in bed a lot and feeling sick. The doctor ordered a blood test. (The pathologist came to the house; I was very glad of that.) The bloods showed anaemia and an under-active thyroid. No wonder she was feeling lousy. But I figured that again the nausea had been caused by the medication, so I took out the Celebrex too. When we took out the Celebrex she was better almost instantly.

Mum was on the antipsychotic Zyprexa for her hallucinations and delusions, but after a while it wasn't helping that much. (I asked the doctor to up the dose, but it didn't make much difference.) It certainly helped a bit at first when small children were infiltrating our domain during the night. Maybe I should not have gone with Zyprexa, I kept thinking, worrying. But when it comes down to it, if you could find something that would knock delusions on the head you'd use it, wouldn't you?

When she became very frail the doctor reviewed her meds. He took her off Aropax (antidepressant), chopped Zyprexa (antipsychotic) in half and deleted Zocor (cholesterol). And at first she was trotting about like her old frenetic self, but it didn't last long and she went frail again within a matter of days.

One day Mum said her eyes were sore so I took her to the doctor. He said she had Dry Eyes and gave us a script for Liquifilm and that was very effective.

It's important to remember that many medications have side effects, especially for frail aged people who may be on other meds already. After at least two disasters I tried to remember to check new meds on the internet for possible side effects. Mum was allergic to an antibiotic, trimethoprim, brand name Alprim. Had I thought of investigating side effects the first time she was prescribed Alprim I would have saved a lot of angst – not to mention public money. She ended up in hospital twice and spent two weeks in a nursing home over her allergy to Alprim.

Sleep disorders

Everybody needs a good night's sleep and people with dementia will have increased confusion without sufficient rest. But sleep problems are common in dementia. People may have trouble falling asleep or wake up in the night, thinking it is time to get up and get dressed.

Over-stimulation, depression, anxiety or physical pain can cause insomnia. The advice is to reduce caffeine drinks, but that was unrealistic for us. Mum would have felt neglected if she did not get her last night cup of tea. It was part of her nightly routine.

The advice on sleep is the same for all people. Try to go to bed at the same time every day. Make sure the bed is comfortable. Make sure the bedroom is restful, not too hot or cold, and is secure from outside noises. Try to soothe stresses before bedtime and give something to look forward to the next day.

Sometimes Mum would feel there were things left undone. She might feel the need to go over the house seeking out her husband or her mother to check on them and say good night before she could settle.

I often read to her at bedtime. I remember when we were reading *Farmer Boy*, a Laura Ingalls Wilder book. Mum was in bed and we laughed over excerpts. In the book a new school teacher had arrived in the Ingalls' district. He was divvied up amongst the community, two weeks per family, and was at risk of being beaten up by his older students. We had a good laugh at his expense and Mum went to sleep happy.

Mostly my mother slept well. At night I left a light on in the house so that she would not be afraid and if she needed to get up she could see where she was going. (Even hospital wards are very dark after lights out.)

I tried to finish the day on a happy note no matter what kind of day we had had. 'Well, we had a good day.' Invariably she picked up on it. 'We had a lovely day!' (If it had not been a particularly good day there might be a pause and then a resigned 'Yes, we had a good day!' And sometimes when it had been a bad day I would say 'We'll start again tomorrow, Mother,' and try and refer to some upcoming event.)

Some nights I read to Mum if she was miserable or troubled. I'd wait to hear sleep-laden breathing then I would creep out. A creaking floorboard would try and give me away, but she would be gone by then.

If she went to bed too early I could be reasonably sure she would get restless and would be out again, looking for television to watch, looking for snacks. If she did get up in the wee hours – which didn't happen that often – I simply took her back to bed. 'Worry about it in the morning, Mum,' and we both went back to sleep. Mostly that worked.

Restless legs syndrome

People with restless legs syndrome (RLS) and other movement disorders have trouble falling asleep and staying asleep.

RLS is a movement disorder, the symptoms of which may include pins and needles, the feeling of crawlies under the skin, an irresistible urge to move the legs and pain in limbs, legs most especially. Of course RLS will make getting to sleep more difficult and the quicker the person falls asleep the less likely they are to be affected by the symptoms.

Some people recommend massage. I found that a cushion or pillow placed under the feet and ankles helped contain the uncomfortable leg movements. But a heat pack – available from the chemist – helped the most. In the cooler months a heat pack rested on the ankles or legs is comforting, relaxes muscles and helps provide a distraction from the unpleasant sensations. In warmer months a bucket of cold water helped cool the feet. Other times I laid a wet washer across her feet when she went to bed.

Note: A heat pack straight from the microwave can be overly hot and may cause discomfort to ageing fragile skin, so I always wrapped the pack in a tea towel or hand towel. Hot water bottles, of course, do the same job but there are safety concerns with hot water bottles. You can be sure that a heat pack will not leak!

Periodic limb movements of sleep

Up to 44 per cent of the population aged 65 or older may have PLMS, which affects their ability to sleep. PLMS is involuntary leg movements, jerks and twitches, made during sleep. Again, try massage and heat packs. A person can go to bed cuddled up to a heat pack on cooler nights. It is very soothing.

- A low dose of a tranquilliser might help with sleep for some people. Sleeping tablets may offer only temporary relief and should, of course, be used with care.
- A CD or the radio turned down low may help the mind still itself long enough for sleep to come.
- A peaceful environment and peace of mind will, ideally, help the person fall asleep and stay asleep for several hours.

Chapter 4
Communication and dementia

Talking to others about the illness

When Mum became ill I didn't know what to say to her friends. It felt disloyal talking about her behind her back, but then her friends loved her. If you love somebody you want to know about illness and dramatic changes.

Many of Mum's friends still lived in the Bega district so there was not day to day contact, but there certainly was contact. I didn't know what to say to them, but one day, Mrs Taylor, a close Bega friend, phoned anyway and Mum rather let the cat out of her own bag. She told Mrs Taylor that we had been down to Bega, had knocked on her door, in fact, but found no one home. Mrs Taylor phoned Nola, another comrade from the farming era, and Nola phoned me.

'Is she on medication? Have her medication checked. It's her medication.' But of course it was not her medication.

'There's not much we can do,' Nola said, 'but at least we can be here at the other end of the phone. We're here for you,' she said. And they certainly were.

There was another friend who did not know. I was going to write to him, but words eluded me. I put it off for too long and suddenly he made an unexpected visit. My sister went out to head him off at the pass. 'Mum has dementia,' she had to say to him straight out. 'Oh, she'll know you,' she said.

Most certainly Mum did know him. She was glad to see him. And he was another point of contact for us both. But I should have written and told him earlier of the illness. It was not fair of me to have just left it.

Should I tell her?

That depends. I used to think why on earth would you tell her? But it largely depends on the age of the person and their role in the family. If your spouse is in his fifties and is diagnosed with early onset dementia, of course that is something you are going to go through together. Other people might be living alone and need to make plans.

But with elderly people who may need some looking after anyway the situation may be quite different. Early on I had organised a home visit from the mental health team at the local hospital, one of my disasters.

Of course Mum asked me why they were there. 'What's wrong with me?' She was upset and puzzled. I said she had some memory loss.

'But there's nothing wrong with my memory!' she said. 'There's nothing wrong with my *memory*. It's my wonky legs that are the trouble!'

So I left it there. What are you going to say when delusions are in full flight? Don't worry, Mum, it's just your dementia?

I couldn't see the point. Had I told her she would not have believed me, thought I was crazy, belittling, patronising. Or she would have believed it and gone into despair. And after a while she would have forgotten even that.

Of course there were times when she did know, the times when she wondered at herself or laughed at herself, so we just laughed away together.

'Nobody told me!'

When we were talking about people closer to home it was a different matter. That was when Mum certainly deserved protection.

My brother-in-law's sister was visiting for a birthday. Naturally Mum asked after her mother. I didn't know what to say.

'Grandma Llewellyn died, Mum.'

'Nobody told me!'

Mum was very upset then and again later, thinking she had put her foot in it. I should have had a stock answer planned for such occasions. I should have just leapt in and said Grandma Llewellyn was fine, she was fine. It was another mistake.

I used to think people who shielded others from deaths were playing God. That was before I was looking after my own mother. If she had forgotten that somebody had died and I told her, then the person had died again for her. Not only that, but in her mind we had not even been considerate enough to let her know in the first place.

'Nobody told me!'

It's both question and accusation, that one.

'She doesn't know me!'

I was lucky that Mum knew me to the end. I know that. A lot of elderly people, by the time they are in institutional care, simply can't remember their families.

You hear people saying: 'I don't know whether to visit Mum or not, whether to take the kids or not. She doesn't even know who we are!' But if they don't visit, who else is going to visit? Memory – and language – can fade in and out or not be there at all, but at least she will have had a visitor. (A photograph album or a book or item of clothing or other memorabilia might help her identify you or herself. At least she would have photos and so forth to pore over.)

Sometimes Mum would forget people and remember them later.

The only comeback I had ever formulated for the infamous and hideous 'who are you and what are you doing in my house?' was thin. I figured even then you make a cup of tea and pretend nothing is wrong. You go out one door and come back through another. 'Mum! Hi! How're you going?'

You introduce yourself with Hello and exit with Goodbye. You just keep on talking. If we don't, nobody else is going to. You show interest. You show consideration. You just keep talking. This new relationship is about her now. It is about us no longer. Now it's our time to give back without condition. You just keep talking.

Communicating with a person with dementia

The most important thing now is to keep the communication channels open. In the home setting there is always something that promotes communication.

When one of my cats was sick with kidney and liver failure I told Mum all about it, of course. 'Not long,' the vet had told me. 'Maybe a few months.'

'Poor Toby! Maybe he will outdo them,' Mum said.

'Maybe he'll defy science?'

'Yes. Maybe he'll prove them wrong.'

But it seemed no time before the end came for Toby. I was keeping him alive for my own sake so I called the vet to finish it. Mum stayed inside while Cam (nephew) and I buried Toby in the azalea garden in front of the house. On Cam's lead we sang 'For He's a Jolly Good Fellow' for him, no doubt to the amusement of people passing by.

'Alright?' Mum asked when I went back in. 'You did the right thing. It was the only thing you could do.'

On dull days we worked out the words to some of the old songs, 'The Road to Gundagai' or 'I'll be Seeing You'. But mostly she would not join in. 'I don't feel like singing.' Mum used to sing all the time, but now she had become too busy.

Things happening in the neighbourhood generated interest. A refuge for young people had opened around the corner from us. The youngest was only nine. He seemed to have a lot of problems with going to school. The adolescents tried to look after him. We passed him often and talked about him just as often. I told Mum that one of the nephews had thoughts of adopting him. 'Ah, the dear little bloke!'

The news from the outside world promoted communication.

Boxing Day 2004 Mum was lying abed when I heard some news snippet that heralded disaster. I thought it was the Sydney to Hobart for a moment, but it was the earthquake. I went straight in to her. 'There has been a bloody great earthquake off Indonesia, Mother!'

We watched and watched it on Sky News. The numbers of dead doubled and tripled before we could turn around.

Going to bed that night I made a poor joke about the tsunamis and the Indonesian cats not saying their prayers. She was laughing again. 'I'm not sure how people would take that!'

'They are calling for money, Mother. I'll rehash the bills and see if we can put in our twenty dollars.'

'Oh yes. Surely we can spare twenty dollars.'

The crews of Japanese, German, Argentine and Israeli helpers unloading their transports – it broke the heart. All the stories broke both our hearts open and we watched and watched it all on cable TV. She expected to be able to watch it.

But one morning, after she had made comment on the tsunamis, she said: 'We'd better look up the times of the trains.' She thought we were stuck in Katoomba again. No matter what else was happening Dementia would lean over her shoulder, hiding her away. When he leaned off she was perfectly normal again.

There were some things I protected her from. But you can't protect people from everything. In the evenings we watched television. There was a spate of cruelty to animals. We watched footage on the ABC News of a kitten being tortured at a railway station. The item had come with a warning. It was pretty horrible too.

'Appalling!' Mum flared up. Mum, who never particularly liked cats. 'What's the matter with people?' She said capital punishment had things going for it.

'A bit excessive, Mother?'

'Oh, I don't know!'

But if there was a new social issue occupying the air waves it did not necessarily interest her now. I might be ranting away, trying to involve her. 'You may be right,' she would say, her standard answer when she couldn't be bothered involving herself.

Other times she formed obsessions and the obsessions became new fodder for despair. She was very sorry for Schapelle Corby.

'It's so depressing.'

'No, it's not depressing,' I would say. 'It's outrageous and a little bit frightening, but it's not *depressing*.'

There would be no protecting her from that. Schapelle rated highly on all TV stations. On the day of the sentencing we finished the book we were reading. Then we put the TV on and watched the sentencing on Sky News. 'Twenty years!' Mum flared up. 'The poor little thing – even if she did do it!'

That was pretty numbing and Mum embellished it a bit. In fact, she was a bit miserable all that day. On a scale? About a six. Six was okay. A six could go either way.

We went to the supermarket that afternoon and she talked with the checkout operator. Then I wheeled her all the way around the block. Parts of the hill path were very rickety. I was holding Mum in place with one hand, pushing the wheelchair with my body.

That night she was off the scale again fussing about Schapelle and everything else she could conjure up, putting everything into one great miserable lump. Do you think So-and-So's alright? I suppose we'd hear. Do you think they're alright on the farm? Should we phone? But who would we phone?

I searched for ways to intercept the bleak thoughts, with something to do or a change of scene. She was obsessed with Schapelle and wanted to watch the news over and over as if loyalty would change the outcome. After a while I turned it off and quickly put on one of her favourite videos, *Scotland the Brave*. That was better.

'Ah!' Her favourite performer was the tenor, Greg Moore. 'A special young man. A special voice.'

When the news came through about the bombs in London I put on a *Little House on the Prairie* tape hoping yet again to stave off delusions. We caught the tail end of the bulletin, something was 'being contained'. Yellow coated police seemed to be all over the screen. Then on *The 7.30 Report* they said there was a bomb on a bus and power surges or something else in the tube stations. It looked like chaos. My sister came over and the three of us watched and watched it. The ABC ran the story non-stop.

I goaded Mum into dictating a line of condolence to send to the Queen.

Within a week the bombers had been identified, homegrowns from Yorkshire, James Herriott country.

'Animals!' I said in the direction of the television. Better words were lost on me.

'No, they're not animals,' Mum overtook me. 'You mustn't think of them as animals.'

Then came Hurricane Katrina. Again, we watched it all on Sky News. There were thousands of people in need of repatriation. 'It's frustrating, Mother. I wish we were over there. We could take some people.'

'Yes, we could put them out the back. Rock would have to move his computers!'

One man had been separated from his mother. His mum had dementia. She had been carted off somewhere without him. He didn't even know where she was.

We looked at this poor man, despair written all over him.

'We're lucky, Mother,' I said.

'Very.'

And after that it was Bali again. The news reports showed children in hospital, Indonesians and Japanese tourists crying for help, bloodied people crying in the dark.

'Jeez, Mum! What do they think, these people, when they are watching what they've done, the egocentric bastards behind it all?'

'Who knows what they are thinking?' she said.

Things in the family generated discussion. I remember when

Alexander (Rock) was doing the HSC. The results came through and he had the marks he needed to get into the uni course he wanted.

'Oh! Well done, darling!' Mum praised him when he came to see us. 'Congratulations!' When he had gone she turned to me: 'Phew! That's a relief!'

One night we watched a disaster film together on television. It was very long. 'I have to go to bed,' she finally said. 'You can tell me what happened to them in the morning.'

The next morning she had remembered. 'Did you finish it?'

'The film? Yes. A great whack of the American coast fell into the sea. And all the other people who thought they'd lost somebody were reunited. It wasn't very good, was it?'

'Not very!' She laughed.

The days when we watched movies together were largely gone, but there were other programs we could still watch together that generated interest. We watched *Australian Story* together. There was a young man, a surfer, on one night, Corby Something, who said his mother had had a heroin addiction. When he was fourteen he had gone into the lounge room to ask her to not shoot up and her newest boyfriend had pulled a baseball bat on him.

Mum was watching. 'Some mother!' she erupted. 'She may as well have been the one with the bat!' Five seconds later she wanted to go home, no doubt to see her own mother.

The thing about communication is to just keep talking. It doesn't really matter what about. There was a time Mum decided she needed a job. Sometimes she would ask the checkout operators how much training you needed to work at Coles. But it became a new joke between us.

'If you had a job I'd have to come with you to take you about,' I'd say.

She would double up laughing and impersonate the prospective employer: '"Who's that girl pushing your wheelchair?" That's my daughter. She's my carer!'

Mum and I still shared some secrets, but not gossip. She would forget who had recently been divorced and other things she should not mention, but that is just regrettable. There is an old ad – I don't know what the ad is for – with a family seated at their table eating dinner. The little boy says: 'Pass the potatoes, Dad.' And the ancient Grandma pipes up: 'He's not your Dad. We never knew who your Dad was!' before continuing to plough into her dinner. That was what happened with Mum. She would mix people up and give the wrong person the gossip about them. (That was a great big loss.)

- **When talking with a person with dementia learn to keep it simple, but not so simple that the relationship you once had is overlooked or overly diluted.**
- **Try and leave out double meanings and vague or abstract debate.**
- **Talk about anything, including what is happening in your own life.**
- **People say try to leave out 'do you remember'. But you will say it and she will say it to you when you least expect it.**
- **Don't make jokes that are going to go over her head. She will feel excluded or shown up.**
- **Approach from the front and with ease to give the person time for recognition.**
- **Use Hello and Goodbye.**
- **Identify yourself by name and use her name.**
- **If the person forgets you, remember that it may be a temporary lapse in memory. You might try leaving the room, changing an item of clothing and coming back in. 'Hi, Mum! How have you been?'**

Memory

Mum could not remember that the other family members had died, but amazingly in other respects the memory held firm and I'm sure that was because she remained in the household, part of the family.

Rodney (builder and family friend) was doing work for my sister one day and drove up in his new gee whiz truck. Mum saw him go down the drive.

'Who was that?' She swung around to me.

'Mr Bird.'

'Who?'

'Rodney Bird.'

'Who? Oh, Rodney! Oh, I wonder how he's going. We haven't seen Rodney for ages. He's a very reliable young man.'

I was glad that she hadn't forgotten Rodney. Some years earlier he had done work on our house. He had absolutely transformed our wreck of a bathroom.

'He's very good at what he does,' she went on. 'You can be sure if Rodney gives you advice ...'

'It's sound?'

'Yes.'

Later she wanted to go home, but Rodney was parked in the drive. 'We can't get past the truck right now, Mum. We'll wait till Rodney moves the truck.' By the time he had left Mum had become ensconced in her picture books[4] and had gone beyond the delusion.

In May 2005 Kylie Minogue was diagnosed with breast cancer. Mum said: 'Kylie. They call her "the singing budgie", don't they?' I was amazed she would have known that least of all remembered it now! I said that was what they used to call her.

That September Andrew Denton interviewed Mark Latham. Mum wanted to go to bed, so I taped it for her and played it back the next day.

'That's not Simon Crean, is it?' she said.

'Mark Latham.'

'What happened to Simon?'

'Ousted by Mark Latham.'

'Oh, that's a shame. Stupid! Political family. Long history ...'

She sat glued to the Mark Latham interview. 'Spineless!' she

---

[4] She was still making picture books then.

muttered at intervals. 'Coward!' At the end she went in for the kill: 'He's a disgrace!'

I decided there were not many people that Mum did forget. But those deceased – the spectres – took precedence over the living. Maybe that was it.

One weekend we went to my brother Paul's place for another birthday party. Paul came to pick us up and drove us to one of the remaining patches of grass where plovers had a brood of chicks.

'Can you see them, Mum?' he said.

'I can see the parents. Oh, yes!'

Beck, a childhood friend of my nieces, rocked up for the party, looking tall and thin and pretty. Mum seemed to not remember her and that was very sad. Beck used to overnight at our place with the other kids when they were young. It's all leaking away on her, I thought, leaving me alone.

The next day she remembered. 'Who was that girl at the party last night?'

'Beck.'

'I wonder if the girls ever see anything of the other Rebecca. You know, the Beck they grew up with.'

'That was her.'

'That was Beck? Good Lord! I didn't recognise her! She looks well.'

My parents' last paid job was at a children's home in Goulburn, where Mum worked at her usual do or die speed. Mum loved the children and worked very hard for them. She rarely talked about her times at Goulburn now. I don't think she forgot them. Goulburn certainly did not infiltrate the delusional haunts, but that did not mean she had forgotten Goulburn. In fact, once when reminiscing she said she had showed off Carly, as her first grandchild, to a friend there. 'Isn't she the most perfect specimen?' she remembered having said. She said the person had agreed: 'She certainly is the most beautiful baby.'

Reminiscing

Researcher Jacqueline Sherry interviewed sixty people including residents of the Lucan Care Weroona Nursing Home, a high dependency aged care facility, for a life stories publication.

'Reminiscing is incredibly valuable,' Sherry said, 'because it allows for reflection and sharing with others, keeping people strong and connected. Since dementia sufferers tend to lose their short-term memory first, they can often vividly describe events from the distant past.'

Long weekends were always long for us now, everything all shut up. At Easter 2004 we sat down and I invited Mum to rummage through old photograph albums. She didn't really want to. I had to press her. I found that her long-term memory was accentuated. It seemed to me that more recent memories weren't maintaining a handhold and the older ones – some of them very old – were pushing their way through.

I was able to put names to a lot of people I didn't know from Adam. There was a distinguished looking gentleman with grey wisps and a bow tie.

'Was that one of Grandma's friends?'

'No. That was John Coulter. He was her boss. He owned the shoe shop at Redfern where Mother worked. She seemed to be always working at selling shoes. She must have been working selling nothing else. He was a really nice man. We liked him.'

Mum's long-term memory could do some extraordinary things. When Prince Charles and Camilla were married we watched the service on television. The other Royals were arriving. We picked them out one by one.

'I haven't seen Princess Marina yet,' Mum said. It was the wrong era for Princess Marina.

Another time we were watching *Little House on the Prairie*. The episode was about a lady who staged a mock funeral for herself in order to inspire her negligent adult children to come and see her. 'That's Jennifer Barnes,' Mum said, 'a fine actor. She's an old lady now!'

One night we were watching a history of the airship and she said the Hindenberg always reminded her of John Boy Walton. John Boy was working for a newspaper at the time of the disaster and had to retreat to Walton's Mountain before he could collect his thoughts and write it up.

I remember a mighty thunderstorm one February with very loud thunder that introduced itself first and then built up to an explosion and made the house shudder. Mum said it reminded her of life in Queensland where storms were fierce and she would try to get the cows in early to avoid trailing them in the maelstrom, lightning running along their backs trying to get at her.

Ra and Col were out that morning so I went over to try and give comfort to their dog.

'Is the dog alright?' she asked when I returned. 'He must be frightened. Weren't they dopey to bring the dog here?'

It was raining properly so we were stuck inside again that day, but she occupied herself by drying washing on the oil heater.

In our family Mum was the last of her generation. So I began quizzing her on her early life and making tapes of the conversations, to try and catch the detail that was going to be lost. Of course, some days there would be nothing, or nothing new. We had heard these stories all our lives. Other days there would be gems, things unknown. I got her talking about her childhood.

She was born in Casino, country New South Wales, in 1919. When she was just a baby her father had died in the post-war flu epidemic and her mother had had to retreat to Sydney to find employment, leaving the girls in Casino to be cared for by their grandparents, Grandma and Fa Fa. Mum and her sister, Possy, spent most of their early years in Casino.

'Fa Fa was a fettler on the railway. He'd have to leave early on Monday mornings and my Grandma would get up early and make a flask of boiling hot tea and fill up his tucker box. And I can't help thinking about these fellows today. There's hot canteens and everybody on night shift gets extra warm things.

'Fa Fa worked all the time. He came home on weekends. Sometimes he rode home on a borrowed horse. He'd give us a ride on it, of course, and put it in the backyard to graze. Gran always went crook at him. "Don't let Baby on the horse. She's too little." But I always got my fair share of time with the horse!'

This is the same person who was virtually silent at family gatherings now, the same person who could not remember that her husband had died. But she could describe her own grandfather.

'What was he like?'

'Fa Fa? Oh, he was a *dear* old man! Grandma used to say: "Phyllis, I'll give you threepence if you sit still and stop talking until Fa Fa gets home." I never earned my threepence.'

'They called you Phyllis?' Her middle name.

'Yes. You're not taping this, are you?'

'It's alright, Mother.'

'There was an old German couple living next door. People taunted them a bit, the dreaded Hun. Gran's idea of a German was the big brute of a soldier with the spiked metal helmet pulled down over his eyes. Still, when other kids were cruel to them she would say: "They are just kind old people. They are not the ones who killed Uncle Will and we can't blame them for anything."'

'How old were you?'

'Little. Five or six. Mother would send money up, of course. And sometimes we would go and visit her in the city. Grandma would put us on the steam train with a packed lunch, a packet of iced vo vos – Possy loved iced vo vos – and lots of stern advice about best behaviour and talking to strangers. Mother would meet us at the other end. It was the perfect life really. When Grandma took us on the train to Sydney, which was rare, the train would stop for food but she didn't trust that the food wasn't poisoned after Fa Fa ate a pie that made him sick, "poisoned". Of course, it couldn't have been all the beers he'd put away on top of the pie!'

I asked what things were like for them in the Great Depression.

She and her sister would have been living in Sydney by then with her mother and her new husband, Teddy.

'We were lucky, of course,' she said. 'Both Mother and Teddy kept their jobs. A lot of people didn't! We'd go for walks through the Botanic Gardens and there'd be people there in humpies. People lost their houses. The neighbour on one side was a postal worker so he did well. The poor man on the other side – he had a family and he would be off in the early hours every morning, working, working. You'd hear him go off in his truck. They found it hard.'

In the mornings when the weather was conducive I would take her out onto the front verandah for a cup of tea and there we talked. Again we talked about her past when I could think of the right questions to ask.

As time went on I was always worrying that I had left it too late to get much detail, but that is the extraordinary thing about dementia – her 'long-term' detail was brought forward.

'Uncle Harry was stationed in New Guinea in the war, wasn't he?' (Her brother-in-law.)

'Oh, yes!' She had a momentary think. 'We were worried if he was even being fed and wrote letters,' she said. 'The sensor intercepted our letters and eventually wrote to us direct saying everything was alright with Harry. "Don't worry!"'

'Do you remember the night the Japanese bombed the Harbour?'

'That was the night Maree (cousin) was born.'

'Were you frightened?'

'It was tense, of course, because many people had their children over the Harbour at school. Of course we didn't know anything about it until the next day when it was in the papers. "Attack is imminent. Turn off all your lights. Get the children into bed early. An Air Raid officer will come and knock on your door. Don't be afraid. It's only an air raid officer." People were very afraid. I didn't know enough to be scared. I was a Spotter up on top of the Water Board Building and was having enough trouble keeping everything in sight! There were a few planes, funny little things. But we were at work [the night of the bombing].'

Then it started getting convoluted. 'I had a boyfriend in the industry. I was always afraid [the Japanese] would drop a bomb on him, on the [aircraft] factory where he worked. They didn't, of course! I didn't blame the government for taking the country to war. War is an ugly word and struck fear in the hearts of everyone. But we were stuck. No good pretending we weren't afraid! We were told one little boy and a midshipmen in the navy were killed. The rest we were never told. They were wise to keep it to themselves. Can you imagine ...'

'The mass exodus from Sydney?'

'*Yes*. I *was* scared. I didn't know what to do. People didn't know what to do. Some fled to the Blue Mountains. I figured if the Japs did invade you'd be better off in the city. People were always saying, "if a bomb dropped in your front yard what would you do?" "I'd put it out!" I'd say. How naïve we were!'

She became animated. 'My mother! Typical Mother! Instead of sitting down and wringing her hands she joined an organisation, which kept her busy. She was doing lots of war work. Nobody else had their mother doing factory work, war work! Church services were always full. The papers and news reels were always of the war. During D Day there were updates every five minutes.'

I asked her where she was when the *Sydney* went down.

'I was working at Marcus Clark's,' she said, as quick as a wink.

'Were you selling shoes too?'

'I sold everything!'

'Did you know anybody on the *Sydney*?'

'Not personally. But I worked with girls who did. It was awful working with girls who had someone in the front line. I don't know why they couldn't get the telegram until the end of the day. They still had to finish their shift. Miss McCarroll (the supervisor) was very good to them. She was very nice to the girls who had lost someone close to them. There were about fifteen of us and some of them were so young. Little Doris. She was like a little girl. But she had some brains. Her brother went down with the *Sydney*. What an awful time! What happened to one of us happened to all.'

One night we stayed up late to watch *Jaws* again. (She was ill by then.) When I was helping her to bed we dissected it again.

'It's probably the best scary film ever made, isn't it?' I said.

'It holds the suspense right to the end.'

'Unlike so many that are simply gory?'

'Yes. We saw it first at the movies. Do you remember?' She was all lit up.

'I had just done the HSC,' I said.

'And do you remember what we did afterwards?' *she* quizzed *me*.

'We went to the Cahill's Restaurant for dinner and ended up with strawberries and cream.'

'Yes," she said, laughing. 'We were too churned up to eat anything else!'

Awareness

Christine Bryden has written and talked extensively about her dementia. 'The myths and fears about dementia – the stereotype of someone in the later stages of the diseases that cause dementia – give rise to stigma which isolates us,' Bryden wrote in *Dancing with Dementia*. 'You say we do not remember, so we cannot understand. We do not know, so it is okay to distance yourself from us. And you treat us with fear and dread. We cannot work, we cannot drive, we cannot contribute to society. I am watched carefully for signs of odd words or behaviour, my opinion is no longer sought, and I am thought to lack insight, so it does not matter that I am excluded.' She then went on to the double whammy. 'But if I do have insight, and can speak clearly or write about my experiences, then I am said to lack credibility as a true representative of people with dementia.'[5]

I've said before that I found that some people talked about Mum or over her as if she wasn't there, as if all of a sudden she could no longer hear. I wished they would not do that. They seemed to think that I was hard pressed. And then sometimes I found myself going along with it. I found myself answering their questions, again as if Mum was not there. It was not right. Nor was it sensible. Mum still had awareness.

There were some things she had muddled.

'How was church?' she asked me one Sunday. (I had been at her side all morning as usual.)

'I don't go to church, Mum!' I said.

She had me confused with my sister. It was one of the rare times she had us mixed up. She also mixed my sister's sons. She called Cam by his name. But Nick also became Cam. Cam did not become Nick. There were just two boys with the same name now.

Every time we sat out the front of our house she looked at a young wattle that had grown beyond the wires. 'If that falls we'll be in trouble. Next time the young man comes to mow the lawn get a quote for cutting down that tree.'

'Right-o,' I would agree.

I found that she saw and heard things *specifically* now. 'I wish that dog would quiet down,' she might say. I'd stop to listen. Sure enough, there was a dog yapping in the distance. Another time we were watching *Little House on the Prairie* yet again. 'Ma has been sweeping the same part of that floor for the last five minutes.' I thought about it. Yes, she had.

Sometimes, I thought, if not for the frailty you would not know. One night she choked on a tablet. I was helping her to bed and doling out her night medication but one of the tablets caught in her throat, one of the big ones, a Caltrate, I think. 'It's stuck,' she said, and then started choking. So there were some minutes of horror.

When I called the ambulance the operator said not to hit her on

---

[5] Bryden, *op.cit.*, p. 40.

the back. I wasn't going to hit her on the back! By then Mum was trying to get the tablet out with her fingers and the action of that made her heave, I think, and she threw it up. By the time the ambos arrived she was breathing alright again and talking, making jokes even.

'I thought I was a gonna!' she said to the young bloke. He listened to her breathing, checked her BP and said to me in jest: 'If she's choking, you can always give her a good whack on the back!' She apologised for calling them out, so normal, old and frail – about a thousand years old – but normal. She told them a story about the Queen Mother getting a fish bone caught in her throat and being carted off to hospital, 'the poor old chook'. The young men looked at her as if they didn't know the Queen had had a mother!

After everybody had gone I wheeled her out to the lounge room, rugged her up against the autumn chillies, got her a cup of tea and asprin for her sore throat and put on a *Vicar of Dibley* tape. I stopped giving her the Caltrates after that.

One day I wheeled her over again to an old rose that was growing like a triffid through the trees in the front garden. We hacked up heaps of it, took out a lot of dead wood, leaving behind the strands with buds. We had academic debates as to whether or not we should bite the bullet and saw it off at the bottom, but as it was I had to leave dying limbs cradled tightly mid air by the jasmine.

'What about that bit? It's pretty stringy.' She pointed out lower offending arms of the rose.

'It has buds all over it. Why don't we cut it after flowering?'

'Yes, alright.'

By the time of the Cronulla riots Mum was sick but still she put in her two bobs worth. (I was secretly glad of the riots as a distraction from her illness.)

We were talking about it. All the news commentators were talking about it. The Lebanese-Australian kids had carried out retaliations.

'Why don't we send them home?' Mum took sides.

'They are home, Mum. They were born here.'

'They seem to forget that!'

By then she seemed to be getting up every second night, three-thirty, four-thirty in the morning. We'd make jokes the next day about how unpleasant I could be at that hour.

'Sorry, Mother,' I said one morning. 'I get a bit … impatient … at three o'clock in the morning, don't I?' It wasn't a very good apology, but she was laughing.

'Yes, well, most people would!' she said. 'That's human nature!'

I had hoped she would forget all that, but one night when I was taking her in to bed she said: 'I don't want to make click click noises with my stick because it upsets somebody.' So she did remember. I didn't want her to remember that! And the next day she said: 'I didn't get out of bed last night, did I? I was good.'

'Yes, you were good,' I said, feeling like a cow again. 'You can get up if you want to, Mother!' I said, remembering a brief stay in a nursing home when she was scooted into bed at half past five in the afternoons. 'You're a free agent. You can do what you like!'

For that last Christmas Mum was sick. She had delusions and was upset. But the thing is – and it always was the thing, I comforted myself – in the afternoon she leaned over to me: 'It's good television tonight, *Goodbye, Mr Chips*.' And she was quite right. It was *Goodbye, Mr Chips*. I had forgotten.

Ideas for promoting communication

Family members who live a distance away might try sending regular letters or emails that can be read out and/or make regular communication by phone.

When family live nearby they might try specialised outings which, again, will promote communication:

- Take Mum for a drive to the beach and buy her an ice cream.

- Take her to the duck pond to feed the livestock.
- Take her to a shopping centre for a cup of coffee or a cheeseburger.
- Go to her house and watch a DVD with her. She may talk all the way through it but what would that matter?
- Ask her where she would like to go for an outing.

Such contact from people she has known all her life will make a world of difference.

- **Don't patronise or play the authoritarian. Dementia attacks the memory banks, not the intellect.**
- **Don't underestimate her memory; long-term memories will be brought forward.**
- **Use pets and anything else to generate interest.**
- **Get a voice recorder and do some reminiscing.**
- **Continue to share times good and bad with her, but make sure she understands that you are safe and well.**
- **Remember that she may well be aware of 'getting things wrong'. What does is matter now?**
- **Try and finish everything on a happy note.**
- **Try not to argue. You will never win.**

Chapter 5
The practicalities of caring

Hospital

There were accidents and miscalculations that put Mum in hospital and hospital can be a nightmare for the person with dementia and for their family.

One time there was an old lady in the bed beside Mum who would get distressed easily. 'How about that?' she said constantly. Whether she was happy or miserable the response was the same. 'How about that?' The nurses were lovely to her and just said it back. One time she needed cleaning up and was crying. The nurses told her not to worry. They cleaned her up. 'There you go,' one said. 'All clean again! How about that?'

But it is a mistake for staff to hope that all their patients are going to be grateful. That just isn't going to happen. One time when Mum was in Emergency there was an old lady in the bed next door making a bit of fuss.

'If you're not going to stop that noise no-one's going to come near you,' one of the nurses told her. 'Okay? Stop the noise! What's this? Your nightdress? Pull it down!'

Behaviour modification is not going to work on a person with dementia. (You have to let the noise go over your head.) In fact, I would call that bullying rather than behaviour modification. It showed disrespect. Disrespect promotes agitation, and on it goes.

The last time Mum was in Emergency there was another old lady stretched out as white as the hospital sheets. One of the doctors was bent over her: 'If you can't mobilise we can't send you home! Why won't you try and mobilise? You tell me. How can I send you home if you won't mobilise? You tell me how can I send you home?'

My sister and I gasped to each other. Who says *mobilise* instead of *walk*, especially to an older person? What would you expect this doctor to say if the patient was your mother? 'We can't send you home if you're not walking, Mrs So-and-So. That wouldn't be safe. So let's see if you can walk.' Something like that? (After Mum had been checked out by another doctor my sister leant over to me: 'I'll just *mobilise* outside so I can phone home!')

The mobilising-doctor was scary, frustrated obviously, but scary. She left her patient and went over to the desk muttering 'nursing home, that one!'

But that's what most people would have thought of my mother when she was ill and disabled in hospital. Nursing home, that one! And Mum was not always grateful either. But the difference was that we were usually there beside her bed, explaining to staff, being a presence.

Of course a lot of adult children will be at work and unable to attend. But they should be able to attend. They should be able to get some time off work the same way that people with children in hospital can expect special consideration.

When Mum had to go to hospital I always had hopes of getting some time off myself, but I found quickly that that was an unrealistic hope. Putting in the hours beside somebody's bedside is hard work, but it is best.

It's a shame, I think, that nursing protocols don't include the family more. A person with dementia in hospital *is* much the same as a child in hospital. They need their family. And all you really have to do when she is sick in hospital is reassure. The delusions were bad in Mum at such times. She was like a different person. Doctors and staff automatically assumed she was looked after in care or that she should be in care. For Mum all I could do was put in the hours by her side and reassure. 'You're sick, Mother. Worry about it later. You'll be right!'

There was at least one time when staying would have been infinitely better for me as well. It was April 2003 when Mum had another fall. She ended up in hospital with a bladder infection and broken ribs. I should have known she was sick. I should have twigged when she was being confused and wonky in the body. A couple of times she nearly missed her chair when she went to sit down, but I hadn't thought of a bladder infection. When I left her alone in the lounge room she tripped over the electric cord of our little heater and broke some of her ribs.

On the day of the fall we took her to Emergency. They said her ribs were so thin the breaks hardly showed on the X-ray. They sent her home that day. She had pain, of course, but I thought she was alright. You have to expect pain with broken ribs. But then she started getting sick. (I don't remember whether or not she was on Alprim then.) When she went downhill I thought it must have been the broken ribs, the shock of the fall, whatever. But she just went *out*.

Liz had come for dinner, but Mum was sick and disabled. At one point we were trying to get her back to bed, but we could not move her and ended up lying her on the floor.

I called an ambulance – *they* got her back into bed – and one of the ambos suggested a bladder infection. They took her in and I followed with Liz, but much later – too much later. Mum had told the Emergency doctor – 'a nice young man; a perfect gentleman' – that she lived alone and did everything for herself. They must have been digging out the forms by the time we arrived.

But the next day we were in the hospital. And very bad it was too. Mum was in a four-bed ward, which can be a difficult arrangement for the person with dementia, especially for the nurses trying to care for her. (She disturbed others and there was really no room for us to stay and put in the time outside of visiting hours; we would have been in the road.)

Mum had spilled food and tea all down her little white Johnny coat and she dominated the whole room with babble and arguments. 'Poor things' looks from other ward mates came our way. 'Poor things' smiles at us, the adult children. Mum was talking all sorts of rubbish. She was sick because we had gone for a walk in the rain, she said. We had to mind a bed for somebody, probably one of

Col's colleagues, and so it went.

A nurse took her to the bathroom, leading her by both hands. They seemed to be gone forever and when they came back Mum was in a new green Johnny coat. Ra was flippant for want of any other way to be. 'Here she comes, Her Royal Highness.' So Mum started doing the Royal wave. This old bag of bones who made no sense at all, but could still get cheesed off at the drop of a hat – 'Where are my shoes?' Why do you need your shoes, Mum? 'I just *want* my shoes!' This ancient lady staggering in your general direction and doing the Royal wave. Oh my! This is the thing that happens to others. 'Poor things,' you say yourself, setting them aside, glad to not be them, *very* glad to not be them. Now it was us. Well and truly it was us.

That night they restrained her. She had kept getting out of bed to go to the toilet and so they restrained her.

Nobody phoned to tell me. It was when we went in to see her in the morning she was upset, complaining about the nursing staff that I twigged something was wrong. 'That big fat one, she's a bully. She said "you can't get out of bed" and then I said "we'll see about that" and then they …' So I grabbed somebody and asked had she been difficult. Yes, she had been difficult. They had restrained her 'for her own safety'.

At first you are very clinical about this. It's awful, but oh well, night staff. They are very busy. What could they do? But Mum felt bullied. And then we all felt bullied. They had hurt her broken ribs. The nurse Mum identified only as 'that big fat one' had hurt her broken ribs. She was in hospital because she was sick and in hospital they hurt her broken ribs.

She still had the bladder infection and was feeling the impulse to go to the toilet all the time. She had been calling for me and I didn't know. The patient beside her asked was one of us called Mary. Mum had been calling my nickname 'Merie' all night.

What can you do? I read the Riot Act to her about being difficult for the nurses, to try and get her to tow the line so she'd be safe.

I told her to think of me when she did not know where she was – I'm home, she's in hospital – and left her thinking maybe it would be alright that night. But the straight jacket was still in her top drawer.

I went out and talked to the desk nurse. I said if Mum had problems she was welcome to phone me and I'd be able to calm her down.

'Will you come in and sit with her?' she asked.

'Yes,' I said, 'I'll come in and sit with her.'

Perhaps the angst was payback for my negligence, I thought that night. I looked at all the things that were hers. You are alone in this room with Mum's books, her things. Her shoes are on the floor, her jacket on the lounge. I could put on whatever television I liked. It was lonely. My own things just didn't exist any more. The house was just full of Mum at that moment. It was all her. Everything was her. My stuff, my books, held no interest. I even missed the endless cups of tea I had to make, tea she let go cold. She would forget it and then say: 'Oh, this one's cold, is there any more in the pot?'

After the business with the restraints I read a press release put out by the AMA (Australian Medical Association) that did not say much more than we already knew. 'The patient's needs and rights should always be the first priority when considering applying a restraint – physical or pharmacological.' It may sound unrealistic to some but I think the ideal should be to never use restraints, chemical or otherwise. Chemical restraints – drugging – hide the underlying condition; the person has to detox off them. And physical restraints cause agitation and misery. Had the hospital phoned me that night to come in and sit with Mum I really would not have wanted to, but for Mum, the staff and the other patients in the ward it would have been the best thing to do.

Mum was in hospital for another week. I don't think she was restrained again. But one morning she fainted or fell getting out of bed to go to the toilet. She tried to save herself by grabbing the venetian blinds and sliced open her fingers. When we visited her that morning the doctor had already been and gone leaving her with four stitches in the poor old fingers. We coped with the usual poor humour. An American would sue, we joked, and then there'd be a nation-wide purge of venetian blinds in hospitals.

And the morning after that we went in to find she had been moved to another ward and set up with a heart monitor. The monitor looked like a small bomb that she could activate herself. The young doctors had come up with something new, some new theory as to why Mum fell so easily. The heart monitor was to investigate to see if she deserved a pacemaker. That would account for the falls, they thought, when really what had happened was that I had left her alone for too long and she had gotten up and tripped over the heater.

But Mum had 'settled in' by then and was alright for the rest of her time there. And physically she was improving. It was as if some poison was draining out of her system and you could see who she was again. (Maybe it was Alprim!) The worst had been her calling for me that night and the restraint. But I wondered if these sorts of horrors were reversible. By the time she came home she might have forgotten 'those bloody nurses', but I was worried that the whole experience might have become a new part of her and might have taken her down a bit further.

Over the years there were other falls and infections. Mum was never put in a four bed ward again, but that was probably luck more than organisation. And after that we put in the hours. The doctors always talked to us. We knew what was going on. And Mum knew we were there for her.

- I think it's a mistake for staff to address an elderly patient by their first name. A patient with dementia is going to be increasingly confused in hospital. The use of the surname shows respect and is a means of orientation. It shows difference. In the middle of the night when Mum was troubled and looking for me, for example, she was more likely to understand that she was not at home if nurses addressed her by her proper name. Nobody at home was going to call my mother Mrs Sindel. At home she was just Mum, Mother or Gran.
- Nurses can't be everywhere. It should be the accepted thing that they can call the next of kin to arrange for somebody to come and sit with a patient who is unsettled.
- If English is the second language you can be reasonably sure the patient will switch to their first language now.
- A tiny light like a reading light faced away so as to not disturb other patients may help the person maintain calm during the night.
- Music would be good so long as the person would use headphones.
- For nursing and medical staff – distract and reassure; it's all you can do. The only end product of arguing, ordering and contradicting is fear and outrage. Talk about the person's grandchildren/home/pets. Talk about your own children/home/pets. Distract and reassure; it's the most effective tool you have.

Respite care and emergencies

Tom Valenta, author of *Remember Me, Mrs V.?* wrote: 'When you live with an Alzheimer's sufferer, the grief creeps up on you, millimeter by millimeter, a tiny chunk at a time. You only notice it at odd times, but it's always there. It can come at you at any moment of the day or night and when it arrives, it's like acid seeping into sand.'

In fact, the Alzheimer's Association reports that 70 per cent of caregivers experience low energy levels. One of the things that will dictate your efficacy as a carer will be your ability to look after yourself as well. If you can put aside some time for yourself regularly you will be able to recharge your batteries. This new situation tests all possible human feeling, from grief and loneliness, missing the person who used to be, to depression, stress and irritation.

People used to ask me did I set aside time for myself. I found the ideal of time for myself was yet another unrealistic expectation. But you quickly learn what is important and what is trivial.

Government-subsidised programs have been set up with the purpose of helping people stay in their own homes as long as possible and that includes respite for their carers.

By May 2003 I was getting respite through Community Options. The care worker, Lisa, started coming into the house once a week to give me a break. Lisa would sit and have a cup of tea with Mum or paint her nails. Mum still had some mobility in those days and when she was co-operative enough Lisa would take her out for a cup of coffee.

Some people use their respite time to catch up on sleep. I usually went to the bank, cleaned the house or I'd go over to my sister's house and we'd do yackety-yak. It was a nice little *time off* when I knew that Mum was safe and I didn't have to worry about her.
Residential respite needs an assessment, another thing I never did get around to doing. I used to wonder what if something happened to me. If I tripped over one of the cats and broke my leg what would happen to Mum? Well, if there is a crisis the ambulance will take the both of you to hospital. If there is nobody to care for Mum while you are out of commission a ward social worker will rush through the needed documentation and help access urgent respite for her.

- **Look after your own health. Use respite time to attend to your own medical appointments.**
- **Alternatively, use respite time to catch up with friends.**
- **Try not to worry too much about the future.**
- **Try to take some time to yourself, even if it's only twenty minutes a day to sit quietly and read a book or listen to music.**

Household security

One morning I locked myself out of the house. Mum was still asleep in bed and when I went outside the wind threw the door shut behind me. It was lucky my sister had a spare key. Mum's old hands wouldn't have been able to get the door opened. After that I was more careful. All day long the keys stayed in my pocket.

- **If you need to keep bills or any other material where Mum can't get at them it might be worthwhile investing in a lockable filing cabinet. You could disguise its function by putting a vase of flowers or an ornament on the top of it.**
- **If the person still has a car you might need to hide the car keys in the same way and/or park the car around the corner or somewhere else where she cannot see it. Out of sight, out of mind. You will most likely find that losing her licence is the actual source of sorrow. Maybe you could take her to the RTA and get a photocard made that she can produce in lieu of a driver's licence.**
- **You may find that if she agrees to give away her car to a grandchild, for example, she may later forget and think the car has been stolen. Hiding the car is a good idea. Out of sight, out of mind!**

Diet

I didn't worry too much about a balanced diet. Mum had phases. For a while there every night she wanted custard and fruit.

'Is it custard tonight? Oh, beautiful! Thank you, darling.'

And then she just went off it.

'Mum, you're not eating your custard.'

'I just don't feel like it.'

It was the same with meat. Occasionally she wanted to make a roast, but I would be the one eating it so that was just a waste. One day I bought a tray of lamb cutlets from the supermarket, seven dear wee cutlets. Mum hardly touched hers.

She would usually eat pasta, though, with a little cream, cheese, bacon and capsicum. (She chopped them all, of course.) She would eat some chicken but very little red meat.

My sister arranged for Mum to have Meals on Wheels. But after a while I cancelled the meals down to salads twice a week. Mum wasn't eating the others. She hated the frozen vegetables, though I would re-cook them on our stove. The salads were good, but after a while she was bored with them so I cancelled them too.

In the last year we ate mainly vegetables.

She used to have cereal for breakfast or even as a snack, but in the end cereal was causing her to choke. So I gave her leftover veggies on toast for breakfast instead. Many would call that an unusual breakfast, I suppose, leftover cauliflower cheese on toast, but Mum certainly didn't.

'Oh! My favourite!'

She would always eat veggies or a hash brown or a Chocolate Royale with her cup of tea. So I didn't worry too much about diet. Whatever made her happy!

There is a story of somebody's elderly father catching the eye of the dietician when he was in hospital for a second stroke. All Dad had for dinner was tinned spaghetti and a coddled egg. That was all he wanted. The dietician was not impressed and needed to do a home visit. Dad was extremely poorly and had maybe a year of life left. I think if he wanted a coddled egg and tinned spaghetti for dinner then that was his entitlement. And on the days when Mum fancied veggies, a hash brown, a cup of tea with a chocolate biscuit, that was what I gave her.

Finances

As at 20 March 2011 the Carer Payment (caring for a person 16 years or over) is: $670.90 per fortnight for a single person; $505.70 (each) for a couple. The Carer Allowance is $110 per fortnight.

Most services, including respite care and the Home Modification and Maintenance Service, are government-subsidised. We were entitled to two hours free in-house respite per week (Lisa and Susan). Most charities will help with food and some utilities bills for people in need. Op shops are fantastic for sourcing cheap clothes. (Some have a higher standard than others.)

If finances are limited and you are worried about how you are going to pay for funeral expenses down the track – Centrelink will help with such expenses.

I quickly found that communicating with Mum over money was now a bad idea. In the early days I would foolishly discuss our finances. 'What bills are there?' she would say. 'Give me the bills and I'll go down to the post office and pay them,' she would say. But she lacked the capacity for such things now.

We took her down to the bank to sign a form giving me third party access to her account. That was better. After that I didn't discuss money at all. I would get her to sign withdrawal slips and then I could take out the money to pay the bills myself.

The other problem that nobody wants to face is, what are you going to do when this is over? Well, there is always voluntary work. It may be a good idea to map out where you would like to place yourself in the future. Some employment agencies have entire websites dedicated to voluntary work. It might be worthwhile having a look to see what is available. Voluntary work can be a gentle reintroduction into the workforce and can often lead to paid employment.

In 2001 Ireland introduced the *Carer's Leave Act*, which allowed employed carers to take unpaid leave for a minimum of 13 weeks and maximum of 65 weeks. The carer was then entitled to apply for what the Irish call the Carer's Benefit for the duration. It's a brilliant idea that deserves expansion. The time limit needs to be extended to the duration of the illness. After all, a lot of people would be unable to leave their jobs to care for an aged parent if they could not be assured of getting their old jobs back when the time came. And what are you going to do when the 65 weeks is up and Mum still needs you?

Travelling

I read that you shouldn't take a person with dementia on holiday. The change could increase confusion. But I figured everything depended on the individual and the situation. If you look after Mum at home you can look after her on holiday just as easily and then you both get something out of it. That's how I saw it.

We had been invited to the 150th reunion of our little primary school at Tanja, New South Wales, about five miles down the road from our old farm. We could stay with Mrs Taylor in Bega and Mum could meet up again with her old comrades. So we had few qualms about going.

Col had a six-seater in those days so we all fitted in. Ra and Col in the front – Ra driving – Cameron beside us in the middle. Nick and Rock were folded into the back.

We stopped off at Kiama for sandwiches and a breather. We helped Mum down to the look out but the incline exhausted her. It was very hot and the trek back to the car made her limp and soggy. I watched her anxiously for some minutes. She knew I was watching her. I thought we'd finished her off!

'I'm alright!' she finally said to me with the old quiet dignity, eyes straight ahead, back as straight as a dye.

We reached Bermagui late in the day and drove to Bega 'the old way', passed what used to be our farm at Wapengo, passed what used to be the Taylor farm, passed Nola's *existing* farm at Tanja and then on to Bega. There was nothing to indicate that Mum did not know the old familiar haunts. 'I wonder if Phyllis is still there.' (Another former neighbour.)

We were in Bega by six o'clock. Mrs Taylor must have been shocked at Mum's frailty and about such things as my having to help her to the bathroom, but they still talked. I found myself saying 'don't talk about dead people' a couple of times, but that was about all. We all went outside and just gaped at the mountain view. We watched the colours coming in at sunset and looked for satellites when the dark came on.

The next day was the school reunion. There were changes, of course, but much had remained unchanged, which must have helped. It helped *me*. Our weatherboard school is the library now – but is still there. By then the cold had set in. It was September and I had not anticipated cold weather. I hadn't packed enough warm clothes, but Nola went back to her place and dug out jackets and things for Mum. We stayed into the night for roast dinner. Some people had fires blazing.

The next day we went to see our farm. (The new owners were overseas.) There was a padlocked gate, but we climbed over that easily. We took turns to stay with Mum in the car while others went up to the house. Mum remained cheerful. 'Yes, you go and have a look. I'll be fine.' (She didn't ask where my father was.)

The house was still there. The salt water creek at the bottom of the hill, of course. The dairy had been let go, which is a loss. (Some newcomers keep the old dairies with the split posts for their heritage value.) The slab hay shed was gone. Another loss. The slab shed my father called 'Grandma's Shed' was gone.[6] The bush was still there like a comforter to the land, though some had been bulldozed back. There were some beasts on the flat below what used to be our calf paddock, wide-eyed and suspicious.

On the way home we stayed in a motel in Batemans Bay to break the journey. Mum lost direction a couple of times in the night. I caught her twice trying to go outside in search of the bathroom, but that was about all. The driving was tiring for her, but otherwise she was fine.

- Returning to the locale named in a delusion may help soothe the thinking temporarily. But taking Mum to the cemetery to see Dad's headstone, for example – to show her that he really was gone – would have only caused misery.

[6] 'Grandma's Shed' – my father's joke. When my Grandma visited the farm he would say maybe she would like to sleep in the shed.

Outings

Outings were good medicine for delusions, depression and everything else. In April 2003 we all went to the Royal Easter Show. Ra and Col and the boys followed their tradition by going on the local bus. Mum and I went in a disabled taxi. It cost an arm and a leg, but we did it. Col had borrowed a wheelchair from somewhere and we pushed her around. 'So Mum got to the Show!' we all said.

One June 2005 we went to a Yuletide lunch at the day centre. And it was just wonderful for both of us to be out with other people, although Mum was sure she had spotted relatives there.

'Well, we had a good day, Mother,' I said that night.

'Wasn't it lovely to go out? And fancy seeing Auntie Lorna there.'

We were both feeling thoroughly housebound when we discovered Community Transport. Our first trip was to Carlingford Court shopping centre. They say people with dementia don't necessarily cope with crowded places, but Mum loved them. It was a big relief to get out too, another change of direction for both of us.

The bus arrived smack on 9.30. I was just getting her out the back of the house in the wheelchair when I heard the beep beep beep of the bus reversing. We were wheeling out the front when the driver was walking in. He put down the lift at the back of the bus and beamed Mum up in the wheelchair. I went in the front way and helped her into a seat. (There were only four other people on board for that trip, all of them younger and much more able than Mum. No dementia.) And we were at Carlingford Court in ten minutes in the drop off zone and the driver was beaming Mum down again.

It was infinitely better than watching old tapes of *Little House on the Prairie* and Sky News on TV. And it had great potential. 'If we keep going we'll be able to do all our Christmas shopping there bit by bit and get to know the place,' I said.

'Oh, yes! We'll keep going there!' Mum enjoyed being with

other people. In fact, that first time a young woman brought her friendly little baby over to say g'day.

Also, in the lead up to the outing there had been no delusions. There had been something to look forward to. And the night after the outing she was still happy and relaxed. (After that I tried to make sure that there was always something for her to look forward to.)

Community Transport had some unexpected trips. In the spring we went to Parliament House in the City, another special day. The bus was pretty full when we scrambled on. It was really only when we were with other people that I was fully conscious of the quietness in Mum now. It was the most obvious thing now. It was me doing all the talking to the other people now. Mum would be pretty much self-contained.

I don't know whether or not Mum had been inside Parliament House before. It was magnificent and simple, cedar everywhere and a thick green carpet.

'Eat up big today, Mum!' She ate up big. I think we all did. We ate very well in a room off the Stranger's Restaurant, served by waiters in black attire.

Mum enjoyed shopping centres that had pet shops. She wanted a budgie and we were planning to get her one. Pet's Paradise had tame budgies and the attendant let one crawl up Mum's arm and onto her shoulder. She loved the budgies.

Going out worked the trick. We were suddenly doing well. We were happy. 'Where are we going next?' she always asked when we came home.

Some of the trips were a bit pricey and she would get downcast when I admitted there was nothing for a week or so. 'We'll work in the garden tomorrow,' I would say, but it wasn't enough. She preferred to go out.

Another time we went Christmas shopping with my sister. The Christmas decorations were something new and splendid to the eye.

The next day was Carlingford Court again. The bus was due

out at 12.30 and we shopped until 12.20. We bought gifts and went to Pet's Paradise to fill in the last of the time and watched Border Collie puppies cavorting. I captured one of them and put him on her lap. Mum gripped hold of his fat belly and he sat still for five seconds while she detailed his personality defects for him. 'Isn't he gorgeous though?' She loved going out.

Institutional care

We can't help but assess the idea of institutional care through our own eyes. The fact must be for many people who are frail and ill that their world has become smaller. Even so, we hope institutions will be as comforting as possible.

We should be able to expect that the person in institutional care can still enjoy a reasonable quality of life without being patronised, 'suppressed' or taken for granted, but we know that some institutions have a higher standard than others.

The *Sydney Morning Herald*'s *Good Weekend* once did a feature on Adards, a nursing home in Tasmania that is setting a very high standard.

'For about 10% of Alzheimer's sufferers,' the article said, 'the disease can bring with it distress and even violent behavior. Many general nursing homes deal with such behavior by sedating residents or using physical restraint.'[7]

Adards, founded by Dr John Tooth, takes a completely different approach. The aim of Adards is to deal with the source of the distress caused by dementia and promote an atmosphere of harmony in the institution which is, after all, this person's new home.[8]

'It is possible,' Dr Tooth said, 'that some people with dementia live in a state of almost constant fear. ... The emotions are the last thing to go. A person may not know what has made them feel a certain way – but they do not lose the capacity for grief, and for

---

[7] Derkely, K., 'The Happier Home', *Good Weekend*, 4 September 2004, p. 59.
[8] *ibid*, p. 59.

anger, and for happiness.'[9]

Adards was set up more along the lines of a home than an institution, with camouflaged exits that keep people safe without their knowing they are being 'contained'. In some institutions residents are hustled into bed at a set time. Adards have no set time for bed. If people want to stay up, they stay up.

If somebody has the heebie jeebies a member of staff will take them on an outing and that reintroduces calm.

Some institutions have pets. Pets are good.

Residents may even be *lied* to. Some institutions, including Adards, have fake bus stops where people can sit and wait stress-free for the bus that does not come. The person will eventually get bored and go back inside of their own volition. And so agitation is kept to a minimum.

---

[9] *ibid*, p. 59.

Chapter 6
Life with dementia

Keeping a diary

I kept a diary of our last years together. One of the limitations of the diary, of course, is that it misses the small treasures, the many small jokes and things shared that help constitute intimacy. Conversations aren't recorded. The comments made over news items or television shows or the conversations with other people are simply not recorded. They are sidelined for other things. But it helped describe and track the illness. As time went on, for example, I could see that delusions became more convoluted.

It was about a year before delusions really took her back to the old farm near Bega and after that the farm became an overwhelming feature in the delusions. After all, that's where she would expect to find her husband. Often she thought we were near our farm; not *on* the farm, but nearby. She simply had to get home *to* the farm.

Some parts of the diary are repetitive, but delusions are repetitive.

The diary also recorded what she still knew and understood. Two years in and she still remembers *this* film. Three years and she still identifies *that* politician, and so forth. (Again, I put at least part of her continued awareness down to her being at home and included in the communications of those who'd always known and loved her.)

Perhaps most importantly, the diary shows that even in the end the happier Mum was, the less hope Dementia's hideous companions had of getting a stranglehold over her.

September 2002, The beginnings

Back to September 2002. Mum was home from hospital after having broken her pelvis and I was still wondering what on earth was going to happen. What is it, this dementia? I couldn't see that she was much worse than usual except for the broken pelvis and weary old body.

And then the wanting to go home started. Almost straight away it started. 'How stupid we were to bring all these things here. Come on! Don't just sit there!' She would start wrapping up the children's photographs and odd things in the day's newspaper, and put them in her massive suitcase in readiness for leaving.

Relatives were being recalled from the grave.

'Will you take these medications out to Dad, love (my asprin and things), because I don't know if he's using them or not, but he can't use them if they're in here.'

The miasma had crept over us.

One night she would be in bed whispering secrets to herself or to somebody I could not see. And the next she was puzzling over which house we were in, even which side of the house she was on.

'Do we have to go over and put Ra and Col's lights on?'

'No, Mum we don't have to put their lights on for them.'

'How do you know?'

'Because they're home.'

'Then we'd better go and put their lights on for them.'

She would come good and joke about it. 'Where are we now?' She would start laughing at herself, hand over her mouth as usual.

'Oh dear! I'm terrible, aren't I? Poor Mems!'

But the next night she was wondering why Dad hadn't come in for his dinner, was Grandma alright, and where on earth was Ra? She didn't seem to know that my sister was simply in her own house out the back as usual.

When she was well enough she made it around to a neighbour's place on her walker. I was trying to stop her from going because I didn't know what odd things she would say to the neighbour or even if she could get there. But I let her go off on her own, which amazes me now. She did get there and came back happy about half an hour later.

She was still on lots of Panadeine and Panadol for her (clearly mending) broken pelvis. In the evenings I sat on the end of her bed with Toby, one of my cats, and we watched the television in her room. She seemed peaceful then.

October 2002, Feeling displaced

When Bali was bombed Mum was still spending a lot of time in bed nursing the broken pelvis. We watched the memorial service together on the TV in her room, Toby and I perched on the end of her bed. We listened together to Wendy Matthews singing 'The Day You Went Away'.

'Very sad, Mother.'

'Too sad.'

Bali was everywhere. You couldn't get away from it. A task force of Australian police was being sent over to help.

'I hope your brother doesn't go.'

'They won't be sending Paul, Mum.'

'Oh, I don't know. He's very experienced. He'd be good at that. They could pick his brains.'

'No, Paul won't be going. He has his own station. I think they probably mean federal police.'

'Is Paul state?'

'Yes, he's state.'

'What's the difference?'

'I don't know!'

We had a laugh. But she would change very quickly. That afternoon there was another weird conversation about where we lived. She asked again would her mother be home and then maintained that we only sojourned *here*, that it was daft to buy food and tend the garden here when we went to and fro the other house. That was daft too, packing up and moving all the time when we lived somewhere else, somewhere in the city.

Later that night she told me 'the other house' was really the old house in the inner city, the house where my father had died. 'You must have gotten it confused with this place!' she said.

But Grandma? Grandma wasn't going anywhere. 'I was thinking of inviting Mother to go to Castle Towers with us. You don't mind, do you?'

What do you say? 'Anybody who's around can come to Castle Towers with us.' The more the merrier!

One night I was helping her to bed. 'Do you think Grandma would like a cup of tea?'

'Don't worry about your mother!' I said. 'Don't worry about it!' I was a bit abrupt but she didn't seem to notice. She said she could not understand why her mother did not write. After all, there'd be hell to pay if she didn't write to her.

No, Grandma wasn't going anywhere. I tried talking quietly about Grandma – no raised voices. I asked did she see her. She said she didn't see her, but felt her presence. That's a good way of getting round it, I thought. Even now she was cleverer than me, I thought!

Reality was fading in and out. One morning when she woke she asked straight out do we live here. Somehow that was unexpected. Do we live here? 'We're not lodgers, Mum!' I tried to laugh it off. 'Of course we live here!' And she laughed herself then.

November 2002, Hospital and dead people

The next week Mum had another fall. We had had a bit of a squall about her trotting off into the garden alone. 'You're not safe walking alone,' I said which, of course, did not make her happy. She went out to look at the garden one day and I didn't go with her. I should have gone with her. It wasn't long before I went to check on her anyway and there she was, strewn over the cement path.

So we spent that afternoon in Ryde Hospital. I went with her in the ambulance and the others followed. And we all crowded into the Emergency room, which wasn't really the right thing to do but I honestly didn't care.

You wish you could get in the TARDIS and go back and put yourself between her and the situation. But she was okay, happy even. The nurse looking after her took me aside. 'Is she always like this?' she said. (My brother, Paul, and some of his kids had arrived and Mum had been holding court. Maybe she was happy to have the attention.) I tried to cover up a bit at first, but soon jettisoned that. So it had become public.

When it was time to take Mum home an RN helped walk her out. 'You're going to need help,' she said. 'Everybody needs a bit of help.'

Two days later it was Melbourne Cup. I found it sad now, but still I went through the ritual.

'Which horse do you want, Mum?'

'I don't care, darling,' she said. 'You choose.'

I put some money on Bee Keeper for her and it came in third.

'You're rich, Mother! Forty-five dollars!'

'You keep it,' she said with bright eyes. 'It's yours.' I slipped it into her wallet anyway.

By night-time she had changed location again. She thought we were back on the farm. She wanted to go and see Mrs Taylor and the other friends who were still living in the district.

I tried to set her straight. 'We're in Sydney, Mum. Nowhere near the farm!'

It was a vain attempt but later we had a good laugh about that too. I hadn't seen her laugh like that in weeks. 'Look!' I said. 'Look at my green lounges! Where the green lounges are, I am. When you see the green lounges, think of me. Where you are, I am!' She was still laughing: 'Where are Paul and Dianne?' she said. 'I suppose they're in Wagga!' (My sister-in-law hails from Wagga.)

It was a good joke, and we were going along happily enough, but by the middle of November Grandma was featuring prominently again. Mum divulged her plans to find Grandma. She figured she could go to Farmer's (now Myers) to see if she was there. (Grandma used to work for Farmer's, 'back in the days when the customer could expect service'.) She could always wait outside till knock off time when her mother came out. She thought that was a good plan.

December 2002, The first Christmas

On Christmas Day Mum was happy, chatting, involved. She had a good Christmas and scored all her favourite chocolates and videos. I had bought most of our gifts online. We had nothing for each other, but we had a joke about that in the night.

'It doesn't matter,' she said, laughing, eyes dancing. 'Nobody noticed, did they? Then it doesn't matter.'

January 2003, Dead people and delusions

That summer brought blazing hot days and horrific fires in Canberra. I was in the kitchen. Mum was in the lounge room watching it on TV.

'Merie! Merie!' she called out to me. 'Merie, there's smoke!'

Smoke! I thought. What's she on about now?

'It's the fires on the television,' I called back.

'No, there's smoke!' I went in to her and the room was filling up with smoke. Our little air conditioning unit had burnt out.

'Told you!'

Mum was looking for her mother and others pretty much every night by now. And then one day she started taking her clothes to pieces. She was so quiet about it. I would think she was sitting in her chair happily watching television or deep in contemplation when she was really taking the panels out of her good pink dress. 'All I have to do is extend this part.'

I hid the scissors to save the remainder of her wardrobe.

'Do you know where the scissors are?'

'No, Mum,' I lied.

'Where the Devil have they got to?'

'I don't know, Mum.'

She was pretty troubled one night. She consented to go to bed but was distressed about wanting to go home, not knowing where home was, the street, the house number.

'Where do we live?'

'Number 99, Blah Blah Blah.'

'And what's the name of this street, where are we now?'

'Number 99, Blah Blah Blah.'

But how could that be? Are there two addresses with the same name, the same neighbours? She could order a taxi, but what address do you tell the driver? Ra might give her a lift, but where was Ra?

Later that night she conceded that my father had to be dead after all. He would not have let Christmas pass without making contact. (She had said the same thing about her mother.) Still, she looked for him and schemed. Where is he? Where has he put himself?

February 2003, Mum's birthday

For Mum's birthday we went to Old Government House, Parramatta, one of the old haunts. There was a wedding going on in the grounds, although some of the guests seemed to be not particularly happy or not particularly something. There was a little boy, about ten, a lonesome and angry little bloke with secateured hair like Bart Simpson. He was mucking up a bit, just a bit, getting into minor stoushes with other kids and coming off second best. Suddenly this skinny woman came blazing over to him and started hitting him about the head. 'If you ruin tonight I'm gunna rip your head off!' she bellowed over him. Whatever 'tonight' was, Mum didn't seem to notice, which was not at all like her but was just as well.

Anyway, she had a good day at Old Government House, a good birthday. The old buildings were her favourites and familiar ground to her. We had a brilliant guide too who showed us some secrets. We had afternoon tea in what used to be the soldier's residence. She was fine that day, no delusions.

Mum was alright generally though The People, the spectres, were on the move. One day she was asking after Neil. She had forgotten. My brother, Neil, had died from a cardiac arrest right in front of Mum. She couldn't remember. Now she was lamenting how he never let us know when he would be in. It was hard on Paul, she said.

When I was helping her to bed that night her thoughts were still on my father and all those missing. As I say, reality dropped in and out. Pretty sad it was too sometimes.

'They're all dead after all, aren't they?' she said in a quiet voice that night.

'Yes, Mum, they're all gone.'

'I thought so.'

March 2003, The war in Iraq

The prelude to the war in Iraq highlighted the major changes. In different times Mum would have talked about nothing but the war. She would have all the players sized up. Maybe I should have talked more about the war. 'Do you believe this stuff about weapons of mass destruction, Mum?' Maybe I should have said it. But I didn't want to frighten her. Most especially, I didn't want her to be seen to not understand. I should have said it. She would have understood.

When the war began we were given blow by blow descriptions and repeats of the blow by blow descriptions. Some commentaries were less carefully edited than others. There was an interview with a young American marine, a cheerful young man. He said: 'You know, every time we bomb'm it's cool because I like explosions and stuff.' Then he added with a bit of sorrow: 'But we don't get to see the explosions.'

Mum was bored with the repetition. 'Oh, not this young man again! I wish he'd say something new!'

'Will there be rationing?' she said. And 'war is terrible'. That was about all.

That was an obvious change. I wondered/hoped that instead of making comment now she was just watching. Maybe she was just watching.

April/May 2003, Hospital again

Throughout all the years I looked after Mum the stays in hospital were easily the worst.

In April she had a bladder infection. She had a bad fall and was in hospital again. That was the time she was restrained and the time she fell and sliced open her fingers. It was ten days before we could bring her home – it had seemed like a lifetime to me.

The District Nurse came to the house to tend the sliced fingers, which mended alright. We could go back to normal and pretend that none of it had happened.

Mother's Day was looming. She wanted to buy a present for Grandma. 'Is there enough money to buy Mother a box of chocolates? She might yet turn up.'

What do you say? Nothing. I thought it best to just ignore it. If you bought chocolates for Grandma then Mum would be waiting all Mother's Day to hand them over. There would only be misery at the end of the day when Grandma did not show.

A couple of weeks later Lisa, the respite worker, took her to Cherrybrook for shopping. Mum bought two cakes from Michel's, which we couldn't afford and nobody was going to eat, but that hardly mattered. We were back to normal.

June 2003, Personal care

Walking had become a problem. I phoned PADP to see if we were eligible for a wheelchair. But to be eligible for a PADP wheelchair, it seems, you must need the wheelchair for getting around inside the house as well as outside.

We went to my brother's place for his birthday party and everybody was concerned about her, so frail, so quiet. She had enormous trouble walking with her stick from the car into their house. They thought she was dying. 'I've never seen Gran so quiet before,' they said. But she was still capable of scheming. Money was as tight as a tick just then but Mum still managed to dig up a fifty dollar bill to give to my brother for his birthday gift. She slipped the fifty inside his card. That was very generous of her!

July 2003, More dead people

In July there was a new delusion. One day Mum decided that Mrs Taylor (from Bega on the South Coast) had taken over 'the kids' place' at Frenchs Forest. The Sydney suburb of Frenchs Forest became another delusional haunt but of minor ranking.

She was also looking for Fa Fa, her grandfather. Her grandfather had been here! The list was getting longer.

In July 2003 the memory had taken a dip. Lisa took her for lunch at the shopping centre. Mum had a good time. It was obvious that she had had a good time. She had bought cookies, but soon forgot about them. I felt very sorry for her, but she didn't seem to notice. Then she spied them. 'Oh, we've got cookies! Oh, good!' Cookies and a cup of tea. Well done!

Sometimes she would be confused about what people call spatial tasks, which direction to the toilet, which door you go through. None of those things mattered, of course. I just redirected her. She overheard me joking with Ra one day about putting signs on the bathroom door and was less than impressed.

'You cut that out!'

August 2003, Going home yet again

The second anniversary of my brother's death came and went. Mum did not notice and I certainly didn't draw attention to it.

There was something funny one day. I had set aside a cob of corn for the rabbit's dinner. 'You'll cop it if your father sees you doing that!'

And something not so funny: 'I don't know where my mother is.

Nobody will tell me.'

When I least expected it she would be back on the farm again. One afternoon she was deep in thought. 'What time is it?'

'It's five o'clock.'

'Brian would be milking now.' In other words, my father would be alive again, on our farm again and still milking cows.

One afternoon Cam popped over to see us. When he decided to go home Mum started fussing about him. Would he be alright? He should wait until somebody could give him a lift. The walk from our place to my sister's place would have taken Cam about fifteen seconds, but she thought it was miles. Was she back on the farm too?

'Maybe Cam will be alright to get home by himself if we drop him off at Whittle's Road.'

The lanes leading off the main road were named for the farmers who lived along them, Sindel's Road, Whittle's Road, and so forth. Yes, she was back on the farm.

Finally she changed direction. It was as if some biological safety valve had been released, as if the body can only cope with so much misery.

'I've decided to stay the night here,' she told me. 'And I'm not going in tomorrow. It's not as if they really need me. What are you going to do? Are you going to stay here?'

'Of course, Mother!'

'Right-o.'

The August nights were magnificent, stars glowing through the clouds like sharp eyes. I had taken to getting Mum dressed for sleep in the lounge room where it was warm. I was oiling her skin one night with some lavender moisturiser she was given at Christmas.

'What do we have to do tonight?' she would quiz me.

'Nothing, Mum. We're fine. Nothing at all. All we have to do is lock up. Easy peasy!'

'Oh, that's good.'

Then she had another fall. It was something to do with the

kittens. She had gone out into the hall towards her bedroom and next minute was bellowing that Charlie had jumped on her back and, waving her stick at him, she had fallen.

I rushed out to her. Yet another fall! But she didn't hurt herself. In fact, that time it was her reassuring me. 'I'm alright. I'm alright. Don't worry.'

In the evenings she would be back on her picture books or her lists. The lists gave her a feeling of occupation. She decided it was time to prepare the Christmas menu.

'It's August, Mum!' I said. 'Don't worry about it.'

'Christmas is a big job. You have to prepare.'

She wanted to invite all the spectres, of course. 'I don't know if Poss and Harry will come. Nobody will give me their address. And then there's Mother. I don't know about the old biddies. (Neighbours.) So is it pork or lamb? We never serve pork at Christmas. Maybe it's time for a change.'

We plodded on. We were fine. But in October 2003 Mum had another bladder infection and another fall. She was on Alprim (trimethoprim) for the bladder infection but it wasn't helping at all. In fact she became disabled again, unmovable again, bedridden, and ended up in hospital again.

Everything was wrong. Everything. *Everything.* She had become immobile and I couldn't cope any more. Even I could see that. It didn't make sense. In fact it was absurd! I could not understand how she could be happily sitting in the lounge room chatting over *Inspector Morse* with me one week and the next not even able to get out of bed least of all hold a conversation. Nobody else seemed to understand that either.

There were no injuries from the fall but for ages she had been growing a massive stomach. In hospital the distended stomach was X-rayed. They found a mass. Was it an ovarian cyst? Or was it cancer? Was she dying?

She was in hospital for what seemed like an entire life, waiting for the results of tests and waiting for what-to-do-next decisions. It *was* a cyst. Were they going to operate on the cyst, not operate?

Suddenly there was talk of a nursing home. Nursing home was assumed. After all, she could not even walk any more. It was the last thing in the world I thought would happen. This time – months, years, whatever – would mark her end of days. The end part of our relationship. Why on earth would you hand that over to strangers unless you had to? But now I had to. And so we sat down with the ward social worker, Ra and I, like a pair of zombies and filled out the nursing home application.

There were the expected horrible days when Mum was in hospital with her so different, half disappeared like a giant bird trapped in a hospital Johnny coat again. One day one of the nurses had given her strawberries and they were squashed all down her and over the floor, but they had kept her occupied. I had taken in her Christmas catalogue and tried to get her interested in the pretty things. But I had to try very hard. I felt that I had abandoned her. Even one of the nurses turned to me: 'Are you alright?'

Just when I thought things were never going to get better Mum started cheering up. They drained a litre of stuff off the ovarian cyst and the stomach was quite gone.

She had some hallucinations though they did not seem to worry her. She saw a little boy in the palm tree outside the window and a man somewhere. (Maybe they were reflections in the glass window.) But even then Mum knew she wasn't making sense and she was laughing at herself again. She knew! Of course she knew.

The nurses were lovely to her. They were trying to get her to walk one day.

'Can you stand up tall?'

'Standing up tall sounds so easy,' she said.

One day she was fussing about going home so somebody phoned me, the physio or the OT, I forget which. I talked to her on the phone. 'You're in hospital, Mum. We'll be in to see you soon. You mustn't worry.' And miraculously she calmed down.

Ra took one of the nurses aside and asked if she thought

nursing home was the right thing. 'Oh, yes, without doubt. Without doubt.'

November 2003, The nursing home

In hospital they had drained the cyst and tested that for malignancy. They found none but wanted her transferred to Royal North Shore hospital to be checked by a specialist to see if the cyst should be removed or left. RNS had no bed available for a week so we waited and waited and every day Mum withdrew further into herself. It was a month by then. She even looked different, bird-like and head down, vacant-eyed.

Finally she was transferred to RNS. We went in and found her in a room by herself, stretched out and looking half dead. She's dying, we thought. The family visited her and they also thought it. So she *is* dying.

The next day we were down for a meeting with the doctor and a Clinical Nurse Specialist. We were terrified. But the doctor, seventeen feet tall but as kind and calm as Mother Teresa, said he thought the cyst was benign and that he would not care to operate on her anyway. After all, she is nearly eighty-five. She's an old lady. The operation isn't pleasant. He joked how he could have nipped over to Hornsby in a taxi last week and all of that waiting would have been circumnavigated!

He said she was in pretty good shape. 'Her heart will go for another two years yet!' he said. They must have been able to hear our communal sigh of relief. So she wasn't dying. The nursing home still loomed – that would take some getting used to – but at least we still had her.

The nursing home – ABL – was pretty awful. The Director of Nursing (DON) was un-contactable. That seemed unusual. We went to look at it in the night when staff were thin on the ground. A lady had fallen. Her face was bruising up and she was crying in a corner unattended.

'I don't like it. I don't like the idea of Mum being there. I *can't* put Mum in there!' My sister gave ABL the thumbs down, but at the time there were few alternatives.

Mum was brought into ABL by ambulance the next night. And she was *back*! By some miracle she was herself again. What had happened to take her off the edge of the radar in the first place was still a mystery at that stage, but anyway, she was back now.

We visited night and day. Col went on his way to work. And Mum had come good. There she was, back on her feet, in fact trotting around on her stick with no help and no supervision. The transformation from her in hospital was remarkable.

But she was miserable in ABL. Many of the day workers were salt-of-the-earth types, but the ghost shift took over during the night. Bedtime was five-thirty. Five-thirty! 'They wanted us *in*,' Mum would say from her bed when we visited in the evenings. She was frightened during the night. 'It's dark! I can't see my way to the toilet! I ring for help on the little buzzer thing, but nobody comes.'

Others seemed bored or miserable. There was an old lady with cancer who cried out for ages and nobody came to her. (She was known to the family and my nephew Rock would go in and talk to her. He was very good at that; I wasn't.)

One night there were cries of 'Help! Help!' coming from down the corridor so I went for a look. An Assistant in Nursing (AIN) was tying an old man into his bed. It was about seven-thirty at night. I was clinical again. Maybe they have to do that, I thought. But would they do that to Mum if she kept getting out of bed or if she was stroppy?

Mum wasn't stroppy in ABL. She was just miserable.

'I'm so glad you've come!' she would tell us.

'We always come.'

'Yes, I know you come. But I've been so depressed. I've been going about looking for ways to kill yourself in here! How do you do it?'

'Oh, come on, Pioneering Stock!' my sister said, hidden agenda up sleeve. (We were scheming to bring her home.)

'Oh, I know. I know,' she feigned acceptance. 'It's just how I feel.'

Mum was fit again, and so we just went in and told her we were going to bring her home. She threw her hands up in glee like a little kid.

'Ooooh! You can have another *cat* if I can come home!' (How awful it all was!)

'Four more sleeps!' Ra told her. And then we went home and rearranged the house. My bed was lower than hers so we swapped them around.

Four more sleeps later we went in and tracked down the DON. She was in her office, which was unusual. And so we infiltrated her domain.

'We are taking our mother home,' my sister said, expecting a fuss.

'Who is your mother?' the DON asked, which said it all, I think. She didn't have a clue.

So Mum came home. They had lost her pretty nightie, though she was down for home washing. Ra went and bought her a replacement.

Col came over to see her that night.

'Oh, hello Col, how are you?'

She was so happy to be home, safe and happy again.

I made her the requisite number of cups of tea. We watched television together until about nine o'clock and then she wanted to go to bed. I was pretty nervous. Taking somebody out of nursing home is no small thing. 'If you need anything,' I said, 'just ...'

'I'll ring the bell,' she said. She was laughing. 'I'll ring the bell, and nobody will come!'

I'll come.

Christmas 2003, Illness again

Christmas that year was forty-two degrees. Mum ploughed into her Christmas lunch, but in the afternoon she went odd from the heat and had to lie down for a while.

Later she had her gifts all lined up on her lap, looking happy but small and not opening any of them. She needed help.

She was given all her favourites again and so on Boxing Day it began again.

'Have a chocolate ginger.'

'I don't like chocolate gingers.'

'Can I cut you a slice of mango?'

'No, Mum.'

'How about a Quality Street?'

'Mum! If I want a chocolate I can help myself!'

'That sounds a bit churlish.'

Yes, Mum was back. The sales were on. The footage was on the news. Crowds of people waiting outside Myer's, waiting for the doors to open. Then the doors flew open and everybody ran.

'There's always somebody who falls over, Mother!'

'Yes!'

But it was hardly any time before she was sick again. She had another bladder infection and was on Alprim again. I was frantic that she would end up in hospital again, but after only a few days of my trying to cope at home that was exactly what happened.

She was back in Emergency again, wild-eyed and exhausted again. But then came the miracle. One of the young doctors said he thought it looked like a reaction to medication. It was side effects of the medication Alprim, he said.

But the next morning another Emergency doctor phoned. Very happy, he was. 'I think your mother has Parkinson's disease! We'll get her into a ward so we can start her on PD medication.'

'Parkinson's disease?' I said, with 'are you crazy' in my voice.

I told him how the doctor from yesterday had thought it was an allergic reaction to the Alprim.

'Oh no,' the poor doctor said, quite a bit deflated but entirely dismissive of his comrade's diagnosis. 'She has the classic tremor. I saw her this morning and she was shake shake shake with her hands.'

I tried to explain that Mum normally didn't have the shakes. Oh, no matter, he said. You don't have to shake when you have PD.

That morning I looked up the side effects of Alprim on the net. Blotches on the skin, tremors, rigors, weakness in the limbs. She had all those things. Her muscles would not work. There were blotches all over her, even on her face. That was what was wrong. That was what was wrong this time. That's what was wrong last time and quite possibly the time before that.

Later my brother phoned to see how she was going and I told him the new doctor's diagnosis. 'Parkinson's disease?' he laughed outright. 'Why does everybody experiment on Mum?'

I didn't care. We had finally worked out what was wrong.

January 2004, ICRS and the day centre

During that short stay in hospital I must have said about fifteen times that I figured all the immobility and so forth could be put down to an allergic response to Alprim (trimethoprim). One of the young ward doctors gave me a little smile when she told me they had switched her to Keflex. Still, Mum had been in hospital twice in the last two months and in a ward meeting the staff decided we would be suitable for the ICRS program.

ICRS stood for Innovative Care Rehabilitation Service, a somewhat formidable title. It would mean care workers coming into our house twice a day to help with getting Mum up in the morning, showered and dressed and exercised. And in the early evenings they would return to exercise her again and help her prepare for bed if need be. An occupational therapist and a physiotherapist would visit regularly to oversee the exercise program. The workers would come from the same group that Lisa hailed from.

On paper it sounded alright. It sounded as though I might

actually get some time off. But there would be people everywhere and Mum would despise having strangers shower her. I would slink into Betrayal Syndrome again, and I wondered how the words 'rehabilitation' and 'dementia' fitted together. Moreover, I felt rather pushed into it. Mum had been in hospital too often. All my bells were going off, but still I went along with it. The co-ordinator of the program came to Mum's hospital bed on the afternoon of the sixth. Already Mum was feeling threatened and getting defensive. 'I can shower *myself*!' But still I signed the forms and the program began the next day. Basically, they followed us home.

Three months! It would be a long three months.

When we retrieved Mum from the nursing home I had rather optimistically expected delusions to simply go away. We were just joyous to have her home. And she was so happy to be back. We had fun together again. I was sure delusions would just stay away. And they did for a while.

Then one day she asked about the Bega school bus.

'Have you seen Wes?' Wes drove the local school bus when we were kids.

'Is Wes still driving the bus?'

I just said no.

'Who's driving it now, do you know?'

'No, I don't know,' I said.

So she had started to want to catch the school bus home now, home to our prior life. When I said we were in Sydney, nowhere near the farm and the old bus route, it only caused outrage. All I could do was stick to yes and no answers until the thing had run its course. It would last from half past two to half past four. Then she would be taking her shoes off again, content – or resigned – to stay yet another night in our real house.

The farm delusion became quite convoluted. It was a vicious thing. It was as if Dementia had all bases covered. Mum knew we weren't on the farm, but at the same time thought we were nearby. For a few days in a row she wanted to go out and wait for Wes to go past. He would give her a lift.

'I have to go, darling,' she would suddenly pipe up. 'I have to go home. You don't have to come. I'm going to start walking.'

One day I tried to fob her off with the washing up, but she said I could do the washing up myself.

'Well, we'll make a cake for afternoon tea.'

'I haven't got time to worry about a bloody cake!' It wasn't a good enough distraction so I had to just follow the delusion through.

I followed her out to the courtyard. We sat there for a long time. My sister came out and starting pruning our garden out back. 'Oh, Mum, if only you'd just relax,' she said, snipping away. Mum was raving on and on about Wes driving the bus and picking us up.

'Wes died, Mum.'

She was exasperated with me. 'His *replacement* then!'

We waited and waited for the bus that was not coming.

'There's no bus, Mum. The only bus that goes down our street is the city bus,' I said.

But the compulsion was overwhelming. 'I'll start walking. It's not that far.'

'Where do you think we live? Where do you want to walk to?' It was a stupid question.

'Hanks' place.' Hanks were neighbours at Wapengo.

'The Hanks live in Cronulla now,' I said, again stupidly.

'No, that's just a holiday house.'

'The Hanks sold their farm and retired to Sydney, Mum.'

There was a momentary readjustment in thinking. That did not make sense. After all, the farm is still there isn't it?

'I'll wait at the gate. Somebody we know will go past.'

I finally had her back inside. My sister optimistically thought it was over, but after a fifteen-minute rest it was on again.

'I should have just started walking. It's not that far. I'll take rests.'

Off we went again. I took her trolley this time to reduce her risk of falling. I waited out the front while she leaned on the trolley. I weeded the front garden a bit, waiting and waiting for the ghost bus. Then we staggered back to our courtyard to wait there – at least she could sit down – and eventually it was over. It was not over because logic had set in. It was only over because the body simply could not wait forever for the bus that did not come.

Sometimes I wondered if there was a correlation between the increased decrepitude and the increased confusion that often came on in the afternoon. Or maybe it was just that when she tried so hard to exert herself the frailty became more obvious.

April 2004, Better times

ICRS finished up on the thirtieth of March. Mum had thrown tantrums every time the workers had tried to get her in the shower. Some had put in complaints about her. They had quickly set aside showering and stuck to exercises and conversation instead. There had been lots of tea and conversation. The exercises had made Mum stronger and I figured she would miss the company. There had been some good long talks, but the whole process left me feeling weary. There had been the co-ordinators, the OT, the support workers – it was exhausting. More than anything I had resented the intrusion between us. But they were gone now and we went back to just us again, singing 'Rule Britannia' in the shower, getting ready for the day in our own time. It was good.

I instituted the hands-on method. Hands-on meant watching her like a hawk, leaving nothing to chance. I used to hope for the best, but with hands-on I knew where she was and what she was doing/ contemplating always. I would anticipate. I would pip her at the post. Hands-on, I figured, was the only way to keep her safe and happy. No more falls. No more hospital.

That was the big change. That change brought genuine peace and security. I thought it would make life harder, but it made it a lot easier.

Lisa still came on Thursdays for an hour and a half in the

mornings for my time-out. 'I don't want to do exercises!' Mum would say as soon as Lisa walked in the door. Lisa would do her nails instead. Or they just talked.

We went to the Royal Easter Show again. Ra and Col drove us this time. Mum had a good day, I think. She sat in the wheelchair munching a cob of corn. Going out staved off the black fog until about eight o'clock in the night and then it was approaching bedtime. It was good.

June 2004, Frailty

The 2004 Budget was good for carers. There were supplements (annual payments) of $900 and $600 for carers.

One good thing about ICRS was that we had scored a PADP wheelchair and a comfortable chair. The physio would just say: 'Oh, you need a wheelchair. Next time I'll bring you some wheels.'

The wheelchair was wonderful. One day we were en route to my sister's house when I accidentally bumped into one of her cats. That was funny, though not of course for the cat. She was lying on the cement path smooching in our direction and I thought she would move out of our road. Then came an outraged 'Meow!' She hadn't moved enough! 'Poor Harry!' Mum laughed in answer to the cat's dirty look. We couldn't help but laugh about it.

The wheelchair was very good, though Mum was typically reactionary about getting in it. Only old people used wheelchairs. 'Sometimes kids have to use wheelchairs!' I said.

'Let's go for a walk,' I would say.

'Oh, that thing! I can walk myself!'

Other times she would lament my having to push her. 'It's a lot of work for you. All that pushing is hard. I'm sorry, darling. I'll be better soon.'

'Yes, Mum, you'll be better soon.'

With the wheelchair I could safely get her into the garden too. Mum had loved her garden. I wheeled her out the front one afternoon and we binned dead annuals and lots of jasmine runners that were trying to reclaim the fence. That was fun. That satisfied us both. Then she went a bit odd and said she wanted to go back inside. She was bent up even inside when walking most of the time now, not just in the afternoons. The floor leaned up towards her, with me hauling her along.

But in other respects she was pretty good. One Monday night she went to bed before *Four Corners* came on and I was raving on about it the next morning. *Four Corners* had challenged the RSPCA over the quality of life of caged farm animals. I had used the term battery pigs.

'Battery pigs!' she flared up. 'That's outrageous! We never treated our beasts like that!' There was a pause. 'What happened to *our* pigs?'

'We sold them when we went into bulk milk.'

'Ah, yes. There was no milk for them anymore.'

August 2004, The baby delusion

The baby delusion happened in August 2004, two years in. That was very sad for her and I tried to keep it contained. Rightly or wrongly I just ignored the spectral baby.

The Olympics were on. That was a good distraction. There was usually something to check up on and shout gloriously at the television over. Mum loved the diving. 'Oh, you should have seen the young Chinese man. He was doing so well, and then he just blew it! Poor young man!'

I was taking her around inside the house in the wheelchair now.

The wheelchair became a new set of legs. I think even Mum was getting used to it. That was how old she felt in herself. One of the kittens, Molly, sat on the black cable box on top of the television and watched as the wheels went round. Molly was about as suspicious of the wheelchair as Mum was. It wasn't easy to maneuvre through the doors and passed Mum's bed so I scraped paint work often, but did not care.

I remember when the two year mark came up *I* was feeling exhausted. Dementia was running me ragged. I thought I was running out of petrol. Everything was work. I had insomnia too, which certainly did not help. One afternoon I was contemplating having a nap on the lounge, hoping that Mum would fall asleep in front of the television and then I could nap myself.

'You'll be able to get some rest when I'm gone,' Mum volunteered.

'Where are you going?' I don't even know why I asked.

'Home.'

We plodded on. And it was time for the federal elections. Election Day was a genuine triumph. I wheeled Mum down to the school in the afternoon when everything was quieter. Somebody directed us to the ramp. (I had forgotten by then how much we stood out.) I asked for help and the attendant stayed with us. She said either I could fill out Mum's forms for her or she – the attendant – could fill them out. So I did it. 'How do you want to vote, Mum?' I said. And I filled out the forms accordingly. How triumphant I was! Mum could still vote. Politics had infiltrated most of her thinking in the past and now she was still able to cast her vote.

I thought the baby delusion had gone away, but one day she told Carly she was pregnant, and when we were at the doctor's for a check-up she suddenly started talking about the baby. It was the doctor who put the kybosh on it. She was very depressed and embarrassed then and blamed me for 'interfering'. I didn't mind her blaming me. Rather that than her blaming herself. I didn't talk about it. I tried to get her thinking about other things. But I think I could have handled the baby delusion better. It was a source of misery to her.

The hot days brought on cabin fever again. Mum lamented often about how frail and 'useless' she felt. But when I was helping her into bed one night I hauled her legs around as usual and she started laughing.

'I don't know why I always laugh at that,' she said. 'My stupid legs! Poor Mems!'

'At least you laugh at something,' I said.

'Oh, I'm not such a miserable old creature, am I?' she said still laughing.

It was one of those times when I was wrestling with my own demons. Dementia! If only I could have taken him by the shoulders and put him to one side. 'Just leave us alone for a while! Just leave us alone!'

Mum knew sometimes. She would laugh at herself sometimes. 'Poor Mems!' But she knew I wasn't going to leave her. She knew I never would. She knew she was safe. Those were the main things.

When the Coalition romped back in Mum had hardly anything to say about it. That wasn't the old Mum at all. But now she either was not interested or was worried her words would fail her. Also, the elections were over. They were ancient history. That was an obvious change in how she now saw the world.

In the summer cabin fever was bad. Mum was saying often that she wanted to go into the City, go to the Harbour to shake off the despair. And I wished I could take her.

Instead we depended on small excitements. One day we sponged a lift with Ra who was driving Rock to an exam. (He was doing the HSC.) After that she was despairing again. So I wheeled her down to the shops and we had coffee. She would get frantic in the house sometimes. Coffee in the arcade helped, I think.

That night we watched a postmortem of the Concorde crash and when I put her to bed I was raving on about humans being vilified for being human and getting things wrong.

I made a joke at somebody else's expense. She laughed outright at that, sitting on the edge of her bed in her pink nightie, laughing away.

'You'll come to a bad end!'

'Well, I haven't yet, Mother.'

'One day.'

November 2004, When the carer needs care

One morning I woke up sick. In the night I had thought it was just cold, had tried putting socks on my feet but found my legs were boiling. And so I was sick. I knew it would be hard going. Any other job and you'd be entitled to days off, I whinged, but you are not entitled to days off now. You just want to dose up on asprin and go back to bed. Delusions would make no allowance. I knew that. In fact, when there was something wrong with me delusions would zero in on the malaise. That was something I could be sure of.

Schindler's List was playing on cable TV. I thought I might be able to get Mum to watch it and we could stay inside, but it had become 'too depressing'. At least she remembers it, I said, the film and the spectacle of it. She had remembered.

In the end the day wasn't so bad after all. In the late afternoon I put on *The Australian Women's Weekly* video on Royal visits to Australia. She sat glued to that while I languished on the lounge. So that was something to keep tucked up my sleeve for when delusions were on the horizon.

In the night she was back to animated form. Where's this? Where's that? What's for dinner? Oh good!

After dinner I was settling in for a secret nap. 'Can I have some toast with peanut butter?' So I made her toast and peanut butter. When I took it in she was laughing, hand over mouth. 'You know who we are like? *Mother and Son*! Poor Mems!' she said, laughing away at herself. 'Thank you for the toast!'

The next day was the eleventh of November so we stopped and observed Remembrance Day.

Being sick was lonely, even frightening, at night-time. The choking cough that stole breath. I kept Mum awake. 'Are you alright, love?' she called out more than once. Carly was still with us at that stage and she gave me Ventolin.

'You're getting better,' Mum said after another few days. 'You should have gone to the doctor. It was Carly's Ventolin that did the trick.'

We watched a lot of television, but then we always had. So long as we did other things as well I figured that was fine. I had started taping *Dr Who* as gifts for the nephews for Christmas, vintage Tom Baker. Mum was very generous about it all too, a bit amused. We usually watched George Negus on the ABC. George often talked over his guests. 'Let him speak, George!' Mum would say. Almost always George had some segment we agreed was worth watching. In the evenings when television was boring I put on her favourite videos.

It was the Melbourne Cup again. I went down to the TAB as usual to put all the bets on. I went to the bank and the chemist and here, there and everywhere, but I did it all in time to make it back for the Cup. Carly cleaned up with Makybe Diva and Vinnie Roe. The rest of us bombed, but what did it matter?

Mum was happy, though fed up with her frailty.

'You must be getting sick of this,' she said when I was wheeling her somewhere.

'Oh, we're alright, Old Woman,' I said back. 'It's what I'm paid for.'

'Not enough!' she came back.

The Americans were voting. Mum said she rather hoped George Bush would get back in. And George W. Bush romped back in. 'Oh good!' she lit up. 'I think Bush is thoroughly honest and decent.' We debated that. But when Yasser Arafat was dying she had little to say about that. Once she would have had a lot to say about it.

Some days her legs were like cement stanchions. Where did the cement come from? I figured it was the heat.

Neville, a friendly local, was dying. That was sad, another Digger going and another person in the street who was consistently there. 'Aren't you talking to me?' he would challenge us from behind their camphor laurels.

When Neville died we went in for the afternoon tea. We had to take a deep breath since we didn't know most people there, but they were friendly and helped with the wheelchair, not that I really needed help.

'I'm glad we went.'

'Yes, it's a real loss.'

'I'll miss Neville, Mum. He led the first tank squadron in Papua New Guinea.'

'Oh, did he? I knew he was in the war.'

There were more hot days. It was hard to keep us both occupied inside in the hot hours. One day Mum was worried about being stuck near the farm again and she needed to get going. So when it cooled down I took her down to the shops and bought pizza for tea. In the early evening I took her out onto the front verandah along with her little table and she de-potted the bulbs. 'Well, we did this job just in time,' she said. They were starting to rot. It was cool and calm by then. And we were both cool and calm by then. It was lovely, actually.

There more good days. We all watched the Lindy Chamberlain drama *Through My Eyes*. And that generated a lot of discussion. The four of us – my sister came over teacup in hand as usual – all talked. Mum said: 'I remember the trial. Every day there was some new thing about them in the news, the poor girl.'

December 2004, The third Christmas

We went down to the school for Nick's Christmas concert. That was good. Nick was in the last routine, *Celebrate*. I could see him, but he was on the other side of the stage and Mum couldn't pick him out. He was looking about, but didn't spot us either. Even so, Mum loved it. It was a shame she couldn't identify him, but it was a good show. She did a lot of 'woe is me' or 'woe is the collection of neighbourhood widows' in the afternoon, but I got her interested in her picture books – she was still making her picture books for disadvantaged kids for Christmas.

Carly took a job in Gosford. She came in exhausted but happy enough at night. She had courage, too. She drove her ruined little car to and fro Gosford without a second thought.

But in the middle of December Mum had a minor bladder infection and was on Noroxin. 'I'll have to get the people who run this place to work out how much we owe them.' I took the little table outside again and we wrapped up her picture books in Christmas paper, which took a while.

She had been fine for days but now it was back. The despair was back. She would be staring at the floor, face like burning cement, and it was day after day of going home. One day I distracted her with *Gone with the Wind* – something else to think about – and it was easier after that, though it was back in the nights. I said she should not worry – it always goes away again – and she said I was a patronising little git. But she wasn't being impossible. It was easier to remember how terrifying it would be to not know even where you lived when she wasn't being impossible. (I wished there were as many times when I just said 'okay' to going home as there had been arguments and times that I had resisted. I wished I could take her out. Going out worked a treat.)

It was Christmas again. Christmas had become lonely. What do you do about that? I didn't know what to do about it. I didn't want to end up like Mr Bean sharing cheer with Teddy! Mum had an infinitely more peaceful time of it than I did.

Christmas Eve I wheeled her down to the local church. I think it was meant to be a service for children and Mum felt insulted by it: 'About as much spiritually as a wallaby jumping around a bush! Housekeeping!' That's what she would have said before she became ill. 'Housekeeping!'

'Sorry, Mother! Sorry!' I said, and swore too often on the way home.

'*Language!*'

Wheeling her back into our lounge room I was not watching what I was doing and scraped her elbow on the door. I wrapped it up, but it was right on the elbow. Well done, Mems!

Later that night Col phoned from the car to ask if she wanted to go and see the Christmas lights in Carlingford. She was in bed.

'Is that my mother?' (She still had hopes that Grandma would make contact at Christmas.)

'It's Col phoning to see if you would like to go and see the Christmas lights.'

'That's a nice thought,' she said, and turned over to go back to sleep.

New Year's Eve she wasn't looking for anybody. We waited up together for the fireworks. She was calm and cheerful, waiting. I put on *Last Night of the Proms* as a filler. Midnight came.

'Happy New Year, Mother.'

'Happy New Year, my darling. I hope it's a good one for you.'

'Fond of you I am, Old Woman.'

'Fond of you I am.'

January 2005, The itinerary

In January Mum was still getting over a bladder infection and/or the side effects of the medication, which had set off some bad delusions. The Miseries were bad too. But we plodded on. One night I put on a musical on the Ovation channel by accident. I thought it was going to be the *Edinburgh Tattoo*, but had misread the guide.

'Oh, well, the music is beautiful,' I offered commiserations.

'Yes, that's *The Merry Widow*,' she volunteered. 'We've got that on a roll somewhere.'

I had ditched the second lot of Noroxin because of the hysterical delusions – always going home – and with distractions throughout the week she slowly came back again. A different care worker came – Lisa was on holidays; I'd forgotten – and then Ra found Mum something to do. She brought over paints and brushes and some of her own scrapbooking pages.

'I don't want to do painting!' Mum protested valiantly as usual. But she did do some though with her usual condemnations.

'It's no good!'

'Who says?'

She started an eighteenth birthday card for Rock (Alexander). Mum was back.

I had wondered this time would she come back. Some days had been just hideous, Mum alternating between studying the floorboards and going off or trying to check the study to look for suitcases that she thought she had booked through on the train. There were small moments of respite. It wore itself out. And the nights were usually calm. But the rest of the time had been a bit of a nightmare.

The sixteenth was the day of mourning for victims of the tsunamis. We put on the television and stopped for that, all the familiar and hideous film clips.

It was hot again. I introduced The Itinerary. 'Later we'll go down to Civic and take back videos for Carly.' 'After lunch we'll go out and clean up the courtyard.' That was good.

On hot days I put on videos. One day I put on *Little House on the Prairie,* then *The Waltons, Scotland the Brave, A World at War* – a last ditch attempt – and then Little House again – anything to keep her happy and inside during the hot hours. The Itinerary was good, though, in helping stave off delusions. 'We mustn't forget Carly's videos have to go back. We'll take them down later, when it's cooler, Mum.' It was something to hang on to instead of the malicious thoughts, something to do for somebody else.

In the supermarket we had a running moronic joke going. If there was a good looking man in a nearby aisle I would tell her to drop things. Her standard response to the joke was: 'Now you behave yourself!'

One day a man made a beeline for us. I thought he was going to offer to get things down from the high shelf for us, but it turned out he was even more delusional than Mum. He seemed to think he had God-given powers. 'I will bless you,' he said to her, 'and then you will be able to walk. You won't need the wheelchair anymore.'

Oh blimey! Instantly I had my hands on her shoulders, muttering 'it's alright, it's alright' in her ear. But she didn't seem too worried by him. I think I told him 'no thank you', hands still on her shoulders.

'I bless you,' he said anyway with a kind manner, and, mercifully, went on his way.

'He probably can't help it,' Mum said as we sped into the adjourning aisle. 'I hope he has somebody to look after him.'

I hadn't expected the man's blessings to do us any good, and somewhere along the line I ran over a tiny piece of metal with the wheelchair and punctured a tyre. That was a tragedy. Coping without the wheelchair?

'We're stuffed without the wheelchair.'

'Oh, we'll be alright, darling. I can walk.'

Not very well.

We were hobbled without the wheelchair, though Mum was very good about it. We had to stay inside but I helped her out to the kitchen and she gave me a tutorial on making corn fritters. That kept us occupied.

Col found a bike shop and bought an inner tube and then I remembered again how much time we spent outside the house now that we had the wheelchair. After that we gave the wheelchair a name, 'Weary Dunlop'. Even the respite workers referred to the wheelchair as Weary. He had pride of place in our lives now.

February 2005, Activity and distraction

The middle of February was Mum's birthday again. She had four parties this year. At the day centre they had cake for her. (As usual, she didn't want to go.) On her actual birthday Carly and I took her to dinner at the local Chinese restaurant. I bought her carnations first thing. Liv (niece) phoned her. Ra came in later with chocolates and more carnations. Nick came over and doled out hugs. And Col dropped in after work and sang 'Happy Birthday' to her. We took her to Vaucluse House on the weekend for her birthday outing. In the days leading up to it she asked the expected millions of questions about what would happen next, what time were we expected, who did we have to notify. I said she didn't have to worry about it – we were taking her out – and, of course, she still worried, but when the time came she enjoyed the day.

The next month began with another storm. What a light show it was that night, great fists of electricity striking through the sky. One of the cats was shaking and trying to climb up my legs.

Mum talked to her. 'Poor Molly! It's alright, love. It's only a storm. It'll go away.'

'Count out the lightning strikes, Moll.'

'Yes, Molly, count out the lightning!'

'I know where she'll be soon.'

'Under my bed!'

The safest place in the house.

Charlie, the other cat, was in his element. He sat out with the rain dripping on him and the lightning whizzing about. 'Aaah, Nature!' He finally came back in with a cockroach, which he put in one of Mum's shoes for safekeeping.

'Do you have to do that? I know you're clever, Charlie, but I rather wish you wouldn't. Put it in Mems' shoe!'

The storms hung around. It was the day for Lisa, the respite worker, and she told us a humdinger had been predicted. I had purposefully left the washing up from the previous night as something to do when Lisa left, but then the storm was a big enough distraction in itself.

We could see it and feel it rushing in on us and then the hail was bashing at the windows. We watched the monster until it blew itself out. Halfway in the power went. A tree down the road had fallen, taking the power lines with it and smashing flat a parked car.

There was no power that night, but the boys came over often with candles. Rock brought incense. We were alright, everybody busy and animated. That was when I picked up the *Poldark* book and started reading it out loud. Mum pricked up her ears. 'Keep going!' she said when I slacked off. She was listening.

But what do you do for light? Mum wouldn't be safe without

some light. When everybody else had gone I took all the candles and arranged them in the shower recess. The shower had a pull out door so the cats could not get in and knock them over. That worked, that was good. There was quite a glow coming from the bathroom all night.

In the daylight we went down several times to eyeball the smashed tree and car, all the activity. It looked like a big job replacing the wires and so forth. Blokes everywhere. Distractions everywhere for Mum. High drama. Kids and all kinds of people were still coming out to view the tree and its car-victim.

And back home it took a bit to get the house back into some form of order – washing up everywhere, debris everywhere, candles and candle wax everywhere. That was good.

The new method of keeping Mum happy by keeping her active required increased stick-at-it-ness. I washed up and put the plates on the table for her, she dried, negotiating the table with the wheelchair, and I put away. I used to take the knives and forks into the lounge room in the colander for her to dry at her little table and that was a lot easier, but this was better for her.

'Okay. What are we doing for dinner?'

'Dinner is hours off, Mum!'

'What brand was that tea I bought?'

'I don't know.'

'How much did the groceries cost?'

'I don't know.'

'Well, that's all very well, but I have to balance the budget.'

I had rekindled the monster but it kept her motivated.

When I was helping her to bed that night she said it didn't seem right to sleep in somebody else's sheets. I told her we were home. We're all home. We're always home.

'Yes, it's good to be home in your own bed.'

'We're always home,' I said. She started laughing. The horrid clever moment of lucidity. 'Poor Mems!' She was laughing again. It made me sad, but I knew it would not last long.

When the news came over that Prince Charles had announced his engagement to Camilla I was in the kitchen. Mum was watching it on TV in the lounge room. 'Prince Charles is going to marry Camilla!' she called out. At the time she was excited. 'Well, imagine that! I never thought they'd get married.' After that she went a bit strange about it. She had the players mixed.

'Is Diana dead?'

'Yes, Mum.'

'I can't see this wedding as being anything but a very sad occasion. However, people have to accept Camilla on her own merits,' she said.

That Easter we made egg parcels wrapped in cellophane. Easter Saturday Mrs Horan from next door came in and we exchanged eggs. She had a Lindt rabbit for Mum. Mum thought Mrs Horan from next door was Mrs Taylor from Bega. She kept calling her Betty and asked after the countryside and the Taylor family, but Mrs Horan took it all in good faith and humour.

She didn't not seem too worried about it. 'Is Betty a nice person?' she asked.

'She's a wonderful person!'

At Easter there were also the usual regrets about not getting Mum into the cathedral for church, the only thing she ever really asked for. But we went down and bought hot cross buns and watched *Songs of Praise* and *Hymns of the Forefathers* on TV instead.

That Easter brought Arctic winds. We were headed for the Easter Show and it was cold. I dug out Mum's awful old blue waterproof jacket that had been hanging in the cupboard for years.

'You won't get that wet, will you?'

'No, Mother.'

Then I put it in the washing machine. It dried overnight.

She was up and dressed in dirty trackies at ten to four that morning in readiness for going to the Show.

'What are you doing, Mum?'

'Am I too early?'

In the morning I helped her into tights, (clean) trackies, long sleeved singlet, shirt and cardigan with the awful weatherproof jacket over the top and she was still frozen in the blasts of Arctic wind. But we had taken a blanket and Ra wrapped it all around her. We had a good time at the Show all in all. I always wished we could stay for the fireworks but we could not.

April 2005, Truly splendid outings!

My niece, Liz, came for dinner early in April – 'the little pet' – and stayed the night. The next day she asked Mum where she would like to go for an outing.

'Where would you like to go Grandma? Terrigal? Katoomba? Town?'

'*Town!*'

So in we all went in Liz's little red car. That was a treat for Mum. We wheeled her down to the Strand. There was a lot of poverty, beggars everywhere and one bloke selling *The Big Issue*. The smell of fresh coffee plumed out into the arcade where everybody was rushing passed the impoverished people. We had coffee and her favourite dessert in the Strand Arcade. It was normal. (She remembered and talked fondly of that outing to the end. She embellished it, glued it onto ANZAC Day, but she most certainly remembered it. 'Remember when Liz came to the ANZAC Day March?')

Liz wasn't at the ANZAC March, but we did go to the ANZAC Day March, another good day. It was a 6.30 start and still dark outside. I would never have been able to get Mum into the city on the train by myself. Col wheeled the chair on and off the trains and even then it wasn't easy. The wheels sort of flattened out looking for purchase against the platforms.

The March went from nine till one. Finally the crowd dispersed, but we waited for the Clans to lay their wreaths. I was worried Mum might be too close to the pipers – so loud, so passionate, about sporran level – but she was fine. And that night back at home she watched the news reports over and over.

May 2005, Me and Mum against the world!

In May Carly was moving to Gosford and it would be just me and Mum again. It would take some time to adjust, but we would be fine. I took a risk and told Mum straight out that when Carly finally moved it would be good. She would be settled and so would we be.

There were small things to look forward to. Ra had generously offered to help Liz organise a Nutrimetics party.

'Liz is having a make-up party in Ra's house next week, Mum. We'll go over for that.'

'I don't think I want to go.'

She did not want to do anything anymore. But we did go and she was glad we did. Lizzie made Mum up and she went into the half-asleep relaxation that comes with pampering, like a cat enjoying sunshine on its fur.

It was cooling down again. We started on *The Long Winter*, another Laura Ingalls Wilder book. The Ingalls family was enduring blizzard after blizzard and Mum was so focused on the book she thought it was raining on our house too. I said we would go down to the shops but she was not keen to go!

'I wish it *was* raining!' I said.

'Do we need rain?'

'Badly. But it'll rain again, one day, just not today.'

'Yes.'

When Graham Kennedy died Sky News televised his funeral. Mum was watching it and laughing. I was in the kitchen and could hear her laughing. So I went in and we watched the remainder together, Mum laughing away at the irreverent jokes. She said Graham Kennedy always reminded her of a relative who lived in Melbourne. (She had not forgotten.)

After that we worked in the garden again.

'Well, we did good work today, Mother,' I could say honestly when she was going into bed.

'We had a lovely day!'

June 2005, The Budget

Again the Budget was good for carers. Mum was still perfectly happy to sit through things like Parliament and the Budget just as she always had done. I sat sifting through the 2005 Budget waiting to hear what Peter Costello was going to do about carers. And he said it. Carers would receive the supplements again.

'Yes!' I leapt to my feet, startling the cats. 'We're rich, Mum! We're rich!'

'Are we? Are you? You deserve it,' she said.

By June, however, Mum was on antibiotics for ulcers on her ankles and there were delusions yet again. She had not had delusions for a while and certainly nothing on that scale, but it was back in full force now. Her mother would be worried about her: she had to get home.

I tried everything: 'Who would look after you if you went away? If Grandma or anybody else needed us they would phone us. We've had this house for years. Everybody knows our number. Of course they'd phone us!' It calmed down a bit or was she just scheming?

The next day it was delusions again. When she had to take antibiotics there were usually delusions buzzing like wasps on steroids in the designated zone, usually two o'clock to five o'clock. (The designated zone was getting longer.)

She wanted to go home again, of course. So I did not argue or discuss. I just took her down the street. We paid bills at the post office then I wheeled her over to the supermarket.

'Oh, I haven't got time to go the supermarket! You can do this when I've gone! Can't you push me to the train station?'

It was Campsie this time, not the farm.

'It's too far to push you, Mum.'

'A taxi then!'

Inside the supermarket it was pretty much the same. I asked her would she like hash browns with dinner. She had turned into Blackboard from *Mr Squiggle*. 'Hurry up!' The lure of hash browns was strong, though. 'Yes, alright, but be quick about it.'

'What about some Chocolate Royales?'

'Yes, but hurry!'

Back home she switched location. 'Will you phone Mrs Britten and she'll put us through?' It was the farm again now. Mrs Britten, along with her daughter Nola, had run the local post office. In those days rural areas had local post offices and telephone exchanges. If you needed to make a call you booked it through the exchange.

That one did not last forever. I had to drag out the phone books and pretend to look up phantom numbers, but that was all. I maintained calm. 'I can't find a number for Tanja post office, Mum,' I told her, pretending to look. The small rural post offices are closed now, but I did not say that.

'Poss then.' Her sister.

'Can't find Auntie Poss either.'

Cam came in the late afternoon and seeing him cheered her up. By the night you would not have even known it was there. All the anger and fear had fallen away from her face and she was calm again.

It just fell away. We made dinner and she ate every bit. We watched *Strictly Dancing* which was one of her favourites. After that I turned off the television, put on some Beethoven and we finished the Little House book.

August 2005, Winter

We were doing a lot of reading. We had read Patricia St John's *Star of Light*, a ragged hardcopy she had read to us when we were kids. Mum seemed to like the Little House books best but we had run out.

Alternatively, we could work in the garden. We had a lot of annuals growing in pots out the front on the verandah.

One night Ra and Col had to go to a school thing so we went over to sit with Nick. It was quite a late night for Mum and she was fussing over Nick as if he was a baby again.

'Are the covers on him?' she said every five minutes.

'He's twelve, Mum. He'll be fine.'

'Nonetheless, I think we should check on him.'

Five minutes later came the first of the expected enquiries. 'Have you checked on him?'

I found another Laura Ingalls Wilder book in their shelf and we started on that. It was about Laura's first four years of marriage.

I wondered if things were going over her head, but they certainly weren't. In one part Laura was alone on the farm and five Indians turned up. Mum showed what anybody else would call normal interest and normal understanding. 'That must have been frightening,' she said, 'for a woman to be alone on the farm with Indians everywhere. I suppose there was nothing to worry about.'

I think a lot of people would have been frightened, I said. The Indians had no accountability. The neighbour isn't going to come over and help himself because when your husband gets home he'll go over and take his legs off! Nobody knows the Indians so there's no accountability.

'Yes, I suppose,' she said.

September 2005, Spring

My sister had tried to get us interested in the Ashes. 'You have to watch the cricket, Mems!' So we put it on one night to be patriotic, but I still couldn't work it out. Somebody was out for a duck.

'Do you know what a duck is, Mum?'

'It means the batter has been gotten out before he has gotten any runs.'

Right! We watched for another fifteen minutes. Not much seemed to be happening.

'Will that do, do you think, Mum?'

'What about Les Mis? We haven't watched Les Mis for ages. So I turned off the cricket and put on our tape of *Les Miserables*.

That September Mark Latham was occupying all available space with his diaries.

The Andrew Denton interview was repeated. We sat through it again then I helped her to bed.

'Say goodnight to Andrew for me,' she said.

'Andrew who?' I thought maybe a boyfriend from her antique past had surfaced in her thoughts just as Susan had surfaced in real form.

'Andrew Denton.'

That was unexpected. She was doing a lot of those sorts of things now. But we had been pretty busy – or at least that's what I put it down to. We had gone up to the school one night – Nick had a band concert on. We had gone out on a lot of the Community Transport bus trips. We had been to Carlingford Court and the Fish Markets with a 'mystery drive' down to the Domain, past Mrs Macquarie's Chair, taking in the magnificent Harbour.

The anticipation of going out staved off The Miseries for some days. Everybody needs something to look forward to, some adventure however minor.

October 2005, Other Susan

Lisa left us to take up a new job. That was a loss and a big change for us. I had cut respite down to once a fortnight because our respite day was Wednesday and every other Wednesday we went to Carlingford Court on the bus now.

The new care worker was due, Other Susan. That was pretty nerve racking. Would Mum cope with somebody new? Would I cope? But I liked Other Susan as soon as I saw her. She walked in with an air of common sense and security like a blanket she could haul out on cold days. Mum really liked her. And I left them to it.

November 2005, The mixed bag

Melbourne Cup again. We had extra people so there were a lot of us shouting at the television this year – except for Mum. Mum was very quiet. She was probably scheming about how to get home.

She did not seem at all interested, but later in the week Clarke and Dawe were on *The 7.30 Report* doing a skit on who should lead the ALP, who could get the nation's attention. There was a horse in the lobby called Makybe Diva. 'Ah!' Mum brightened up. 'Very clever.'

Paul and Di came home from their overseas holiday. We made a cake and invited them over for afternoon tea. Paul was very animated. He had not much liked the flight. 'There ought to be etiquette about seating,' he said. 'The bloke in front of you lays his seat back so far you can hardly move. You don't lay your seat back because then you'll squash the poor bugger behind you ...' Mum sat quietly through it all. She seemed to not keep up. But after they had gone she talked about the trip to Britain we had taken years ago. She picked up steam. 'Remember Warwick Castle? Remember the grounds? The peacocks!'

It was time for the twenty-first birthday party of Paul's son, Josh. Mum had trouble with groups by now. Also Lisa came to see Mum that day. We bought her a pot of carnations as a thank you and had tea in the courtyard. And then it was time to get ready for Josh's party. Perhaps it was a bit much, too much to do, too many people.

Josh's party started 3.30 pm. There was extra family there, Di's mother and family, Wayne and Denise. Mum remembered them. Wayne took her frail old hand and gave her a kiss. Yes, she remembered them! Denise was lovely to her, talking with her, *believing* her, though Mum had started getting stroppy. The hours were too long for her. She was coping less.

'Where's my blue cardigan?'

'At home, Mum. It's safe at home.'

'No, no! It's here. I know it's here. I know I brought it with me.'

'It's home, Mum.'

'I tell you it's *here!*'

Denise said they would find it tomorrow when they cleaned up and would set it aside for safekeeping. From six o'clock – even before dinner – Mum was fussing about the spectres. Somebody might be missing us.

'We have to wait for dinner!' I said. 'Aren't you hungry? I'm starved!'

'And Liv is bringing her young man tonight,' Denise added. 'You've got to check him out!'

We did stay for dinner and then Col took us home.

Josh phoned the next day to thank us for our gift so I put Mum on the phone. 'No, Josh isn't here!' she said. Then she realised and I heard her saying. 'Oh, it's you, darling!' She finished the call and called back into me in the living room. 'That was Josh,' she said. 'He's a splendid young man!' she said, all lit up.

In November there was a massive swoop by police of all persuasions on a bunch of people who were thought to be planning terrorist acts here. We watched it over and over on the television.

The spectres were around a fair bit. Mum wanted to buy them Christmas presents.

She was not particularly well. She stayed in bed in the mornings and came to life later in the day.

We missed the day centre's Christmas Party. We were both really looking forward to that, but she had pain and had been sick all week.

We had started on *A Royal Duty*, the Paul Burrell book on Princess Diana. She laid in bed while I read to her.

'Keep going! Lazy bones!'

December 2005, The last Christmas

So Mum was sick again. Her legs had turned into bags of wet cement again. For a few days I wondered if she'd started on the death march. But then the doctor diagnosed a bladder infection and gave her Keflex again.

Even then there were the usual obsessions. The young man Van Nguyen was hanged in Singapore. Mum was very upset about that, but happily on the day she slept in and did not surface until it was all over. After an appropriate amount of watching it on Sky News I turned the television off and we went out into the garden. I gave her branches to chop and she made leaf compost. She used to just chop branches so they would fit more easily into the green bin, but now she wanted to make compost out of everything. But that was alright. Everybody needs a project, I thought, and when it all rots down we'll have good compost. She said – she *still* said – you can't put the compost into the garden before it has properly broken down otherwise you run the risk of introducing moulds and viruses.

That night she was in despair again over Van Nguyen and general loneliness so I dug out our Christmas presents and we started wrapping them up. I said we would wrap two a night, but she wanted to keep going so we wrapped up everything. She was alright again.

I had fear though. It would not go away. Would this be the last Christmas with her? Most likely, I thought. It was two years since she was in ABL. And two years since the doctor in Royal North Shore told us comfortingly – it was comforting then – 'she's in good nick; her heart has another two years in it yet!' Well, it is two years, I said to myself. I just wanted a quiet time with her this Christmas. All my efforts were centred on that.

John Doyle's *Changi* had started on the History channel.

'It breaks the heart, Mother, but I have a vested interest in these old men so I have to watch it.'

'We don't *have* to watch it,' she said, already knowing the answer.

'I feel obliged to watch it.'

'Yes.'

We were talking about the war in the Pacific. 'Well, of course the Japs wanted the same thing as the Americans,' she said. 'They were after the oil!'

She was still unwell. 'Are *you* alright?' she said one morning when I went in to her. Am I alright! I asked how she was. She said her ear was sore and started laughing. Her ankles were sore from

146

the horrible rotten mongrel ulcers. Her hip was sore. She had pains in her stomach. And now she had a sore ear!

'Is your nose sore?' I said. 'Are your eyebrows sore?'

'Only my ear. I was probably sleeping on it!'

I had bought her new clothes for an upcoming birthday party, a new top and trousers. I tried them on her first thing in the morning when she was getting out of bed. The top fitted well and she loved it: 'That's smart,' she said. But the pants didn't fit.

'Too squeezy? Oh, well, I'll see if they fit me. See, I didn't really buy them for you, Mother!' I said.

'I was thinking … but didn't want to say it!' she came back, and then she was laughing.

I tried the pants on in her room: 'They're a bit squeezy on me too, but not too bad,' I said. 'Not like The Big Lady who wears everything two sizes too small and looks as though she has small animals in there trying to escape.'

She doubled up laughing. 'That's exactly what she looks like!' she said.

It was my birthday a few days later and Mum was sick. I had taken her back to the doctor and he had given her Flagyl, but it had made her nauseous. Ra had some Maxolin, thank goodness, and she eventually came good enough to venture out for a couple of hours.

Ron and Susan – the Grandma connection – came for my party. That was good of them, but Mum was not well. She sat in the wheelchair while we did presents. I scored money and some precious things. Lastly I opened a gift from Josh. I could feel a picture frame. He had framed for me a drawing he'd made of my brother Neil when they went on a fishing trip together not long before he died.

'Imagine that!' I said audibly to her. Imagine that the boy would do this and that he would give this priceless thing to me! But in Mum it did not register. Neil was still missing in action. Why make such a fuss?

The next day she had delusions. She was ill and the delusions were bad for her. She was franticly looking for Paul to get him to take her home. I had to wheel her around the neighbourhood looking for Paul and eventually phoned him at his house to get him to talk to her.

'How are you going, Mum?' I could hear him saying to her. 'It's a hot day, isn't it?' The mission had been to locate Paul so she calmed down.

I took her to the kitchen then and we slavishly did the washing up and cleaned out cupboards. That helped.

In the morning I asked the doctor to do a home visit. He gave us more scripts.

I thought she was going to come good, but I was wrong. She was sick again and had pains in her stomach again. I gave her a Maxolin. She was sitting up in the lounge room and watching Little House then. I reverted again too. Maybe she *had* begun the death march after all. It was frightening.

We were booked for the Community Transport Christmas party, which was to be dinner at the RSL and then a drive to look at the Christmas lights. But Mum was sick again. That was the second party we had missed. We normally did not have parties to go to.

It was me doing the miseries now, but at about two-thirty delusions hit. There was comfort in that. I looked after her and worried over her all morning and in the afternoons it was business as usual! The delusion wasn't too bad. I took her out to the courtyard and she chopped privet for a short while.

The next day she came good.

'You're feeling better, aren't you?'

'Yes,' she said, happily.

'Infinitely better?'

'Infinitely better,' she said.

But in a couple of days she had taken to her bed again.

'I've become gloomy, Mother,' I said from her bedside.

'Yes, it's lonely when somebody is sick. I used to hate it when

Mother was sick. Of course Mother was rarely sick. That's probably why she didn't have much tolerance herself.'

The sore hip was paining her. It was hot and swollen so I rushed her down to the doctor again. Bursitis. He gave her a steroid injection. She sat as straight as a dye while he gave her the needle and only complained to me later. 'God, that hurt!'

The next morning she said the hip was no better, but by the afternoon it seemed a little better, less hot and swollen. And then delusions kicked in and she forgot all about the bursitis. We went down the street and posted Christmas cards.

Three days before Christmas we finished the Paul Burrell book. That was one thing. I just raced through the last few pages. We had come to the part where Mr Burrell was in the Old Bailey. He saw the inscription *Honni soit qui mal y pense*. I thought it was Latin.

'It's French!' Mum defeated me. She rattled it off. '*Shame upon him who thinks evil of it.*'

'What does it mean? Don't prejudge?'

'Something like that.'

She still had bouts of pain and nausea. And always, always, always there was the problem of the ulcers on her ankles. I went back to putting the Duoderm patches on them so they were mushy again and more obvious to her than ever. And she had pain.

'Where's the pain, Mum?'

'In my back. Just here. My back is so sore.'

I bought some Dencorub and ladled that in. 'Aah, that's lovely. Thank you.'

I put Christmas decorations throughout her room to cheer it up. 'Oh, that's better!' she said. 'Much better!'

We had finished the Paul Burrell book and needed something else to start on. 'Do you want your Christmas present now?'

'Alright!' She lit up.

I dug out *Little House in the Big Woods*. I hadn't even wrapped it yet.

'Don't tell anybody,' I said.

'I won't tell anybody!'

And we started on that. It was the first in the series. I wanted to get started on it.

Dying

We were going to take Mum in for the cathedral Christmas Eve service, but on the day there was a heat wave. It was a shame, but I didn't think she was up to it, though right into the afternoon I was wondering if we should go or not.

In the night I was looking for Christmas carols on TV, but the best we could find were in *Inspector Poirot*.

'Jeez, Mum! When I was little the ABC played carols all the time. It is Christmas, after all!'

'Everybody played carols.'

We had some Christmas cooking to do. Mum had been enthusiastic about helping, but in the end she stayed in bed. It seemed she had been sick for a thousand years. (I had asked the doctor down again. He mentioned tests, tests that would be best done in hospital.)

Christmas day Mum was up and dressed about midday and I took her into the kitchen. She was happy to help with the washing up. But when it was time to go over for Christmas lunch she didn't want to go. She had the days wrong. She was upset about it.

'I'm not ready! Christmas is tomorrow!'

After lunch she went back to bed and we read *Little House in the Big Woods* again. Then came delusions. 'Would somebody take me home? How am I going to get home?' That was unexpected. It was not comforting this time. She was normally happy on Christmas Day with all the family there. She did communicate with the kids, but all in all she had a miserable last Christmas.

The next day I decided she needed to be in hospital. She was hardly drinking. I figured she must have been dehydrated. And there was still the illness. She needed to be in hospital, the last place on earth I wanted her to be.

'I have been wondering,' she said when I put it to her.

So with the usual trepidation off we went to hospital.

They were very busy because of the Christmas weekend. I had not planned on that. All the medical centres were closed, of course, and the hospital was operating on a skeleton staff.

Mum's blood pressure was through the roof, and so they admitted her. That was a relief. Ra and I went home.

The next day Col gave me a lift to the hospital. Mum was sitting in her chair and watching the door. She was waiting for me and gave me a happy 'oh, there's Mems!' smile. She looked very much better. They had a drip in.

'There you go, Mother,' I said. 'You needed to be dripped.'

'They think I might be home tomorrow.'

She was normal. The food trolley was brought around. 'Is *that* my lunch?' Chicken broth and jelly. I helped her eat and made ready to go home. She was so normal, but it was the beginning of the end. Right there and then she became very ill. She started vomiting and could not stop.

I stayed for a while then left. I was hoping she would sleep, sleep it off. Three hours later we went back and there she was, stretched out like a dying kitten.

She was given oxygen. 'Will you take my glasses off?' The oxygen mask.

'In the morning, Mother, I'll bring in Little House and we'll do some of that.'

'Thank you.'

In the morning she was certainly looking better. The oxygen mask was gone. Her BP was down. And she asked me straight out. 'Did you think I was dying last night?'

In the late afternoon we went home for a while. She's alright, we said. She'll be alright. But then another doctor phoned, Lisa. And there it was. She had found two masses on a scan.

'One would be the ovarian cyst.'

'I don't think it's the cyst.'

She came in when we were in the ward that night. The thing has leaned against the bowel and shut it off. That was what was wrong. She said it was most likely a malignancy, ovarian cancer, but also that she had sent through a note to pathology to please check liver, kidneys and so forth, and the results showed that it hadn't spread. There may be something that can be done about it, we said. Lisa didn't say that, but we said it.

In the morning Mum was transferred to a two-bed ward. She had the window seat again. She said the camphor laurel outside needed pruning.

She was Nil by Mouth, although her new young doctor Nicholas conceded to sips of water. Even that he seemed doubtful about. Her heart was beating too fast, but her blood tests didn't indicate a heart attack. She was down for another ultrasound on Tuesday and then maybe they'll be able to drain the thing, whichever it is. Oh, yes, there was hope!

But in the afternoon four doctors descended on us, the gynae registrar, her associate, Lisa from the day before and a Dr K., an obstets doctor. They shut the door behind them. (Mum was in a deep sleep.) Dr K. was the spokesperson. 'How is Mum's quality of life?' he asked me. No matter what I answered, he was going to modify his words accordingly. They thought she was full of cancer. No, they were sure she was full of cancer otherwise they wouldn't have told us. They wanted the final ultrasound to be sure, but they were sure.

When somebody is dying the last communications with that person become stencilled onto you like a new skin. They become more important than anything else.

Ra and I sat the hours and days beside her. When she was confused they gave her oxygen and she would come back. But she had started to die. She had been offered morphine. The nurses said she was too quiet, uncomplaining, about pain. I told her she must speak up if she had pain. She had pneumonia too. It was bad for her.

'If this is pneumonia, I don't think much of it. They are not overly excited about my progress.'

We talked with the staff about palliative care. But the public holidays were going to hold plans back.

I hated leaving her and I hated staying. I would come home from the hospital and go straight down to the shops again because I couldn't bear the *nothing* in the house. In the nights I would hear her. Half asleep I'd leap out of bed. 'I'm coming!' I would hurry out to reassure shadows.

But there in the hospital Mum was still communicating. The kids would visit her. Liv came in for an embrace. 'Hello, darling!' Mum welcomed her. 'You know, darling, you're going to make a beautiful bride one day,' she told her. The devotion to family never waned.

New Year's Eve we were in the hospital and Mum choked on a tablet. She was *drowning* on it. I pursued nurses. 'She's choking!' Several came in. It took forever. If only she would die and be free of it, I thought. But the body just clings to life. I stayed with her down the bottom of the bed where I wouldn't be in their road while they suctioned her out.

For the next days she lay in a big padded chair while I read out chapters of the Little House book. She smiled at the appropriate places. She looked at the drawing of Laura going off to town. 'Go on,' she said when I slacked off.

I told her how when I was watering the garden I saw Alexander creeping home from New Year's about six o'clock in the morning.

'It's so *normal*, isn't it?' I said.

'It is normal,' she said.

'He's a dear young man.'

'A very decent young man,' she said. (I'm sure we'd said the same of all of the kids on one day or another!)

She was pretty good. Or good enough. And she was talking. 'Do you want a cookie?' to Nick though of course there were no cookies. She still called him Cam. She was still raving on about dead people.

'How is your father?'

'He's good,' my sister said. 'Dad's fine.'

Days were like entire lifetimes. She was very uncomfortable now. The morphine made her words barely audible some days. Her arms were bruised and bloody from the drips. The scar from the day centre accident still shone out amongst them as though it was trying to elbow the others out of the road. You pretend. Old people are brave. They don't have suffering. It doesn't matter! Maybe she doesn't notice, all tucked up in the white and chrome of hospital. Maybe she did not know. Of course she knew.

That last day we were late in. My fault. I had been scrubbing the house in the hope of bringing her home with palliative care. She was just back from the ultrasound looking clean and relaxed.

'You look pretty,' I said.

'You're beautiful!' Whispery, worn old voice.

The public holidays were over and the hospital had come to life again. But Mum had a bad day that last day. It seemed to take ten years to get an injection of morphine. I asked a few times for morphine. They were just busy. And the two-nurse system protocol is slow. (One nurse has to check the dispensation of morphine with another.)

'Don't lean on the window!' she whispered when she caught me staring out.

Rodney is on the mend, Ra told her. (The builder friend had been sick with pneumonia himself.)

'I'm glad he's better,' she said.

Before we left from the afternoon session we talked to her about getting her home. 'You can lie in bed and watch Little House and *Riverdance* and *Les Miserables* and *Scotland the Brave* and *Last Night of the Proms*, all your favourites.'

'*Last Night of the Proms*!'

But in the early evening Dr H., who was now in charge of her, phoned saying that Mum was going down, down, down. She was trying fluids in the hope of picking her up.

And so the dire aloneness was back. There was this great stony chasm just waiting for me to slip into it. How do you cope with it? It crept out of the walls to overcome.

We went back later that night. Mum woke up but didn't really want us there. 'Go home,' she said. That was about 8 o'clock. 'Go home.' Rock gave her a big hug and he said later he could feel her holding onto him.

About eleven o'clock that night another doctor phoned to say that Mum had choked on a tablet again and it would be a good thing to come and sit with her. She had done the drowning again. Col drove me and we stayed with her. She died a bit after midnight.

Epilogue

When we realised that Mum was dying we tried to get her home with palliative care so that she could die in the comfort of her own bed. That was what she wanted. That was what we wanted. But the public holidays delayed everything. We did not get her home in time.

We sat in the hospital and planned her funeral. We planned to have the burial first followed by the church service and the celebration of that long and varied life. That was good. That worked. That was how we had buried our brother. You get the administrative misery out of the way and then you can go on to the celebration of life. It worked.

We were buoyed along by others. Even Dr H. from the hospital phoned Ra the morning after to make sure she knew. She sent her love to the family. She is a special one, but then they all were – the nurses, the assistants, all of them.

When I read over my notes now with some objectivity I have to admit that Mum could be pretty mad sometimes. But that's not how I remember our life together. Of course I remember the batches of delusions – four lots a day when things were really bad. I remember the tantrums she threw sometimes and the tantrums I sometimes threw back. I remember the grief and the guilt. Carer's guilt is like an overcoat made of cement that you try and hide in the back of the wardrobe where nobody can see but, when you least expect it, it wraps itself around your shoulders again. All carers know about the coat made of cement. Heavy it is too. It goes back into the wardrobe leaving me exhausted even now.

Mostly I just think of us. It may seem sentimental or even not at all genuine, but what I think of is us, how close we were, how united we remained, even how much *fun* we had together. As I have said, the diary does not offer up the many small moments that people share together and in that respect it is a flawed instrument.

When Mum died – when the last tortured breath couldn't go in – I thought if you could put both my hands together one hand would be relief, the other sorrow. Relief and sorrow in exact and equal portions. No more suffering – except for here.

Where was she? She was simply gone. Not a shadow or cold fog or anything like that. We will never share anything again. Never touch again. Laugh again. All that history – all that life – is simply gone. You'll never be able to retrieve any of it, I thought. The freight train has borne down and scooped her off with me just standing there stupidly watching, and she is gone.

But now, all this time later, I hear her again. I see her laughing over some aside or some new embarrassing thing that I have done. I see her being kinder than most others still, more understanding than most others, *quicker* than most others. I feel her cold thin hand in mine. I remember.

If somebody were to ask me now how the illness progressed in Mum I would be hard pressed to give a decent answer. I don't know if that was because our last year together was the happiest, and therefore I simply didn't notice dramatic changes, or because changes were actually subtle. I think the latter. I certainly looked for changes. There were batches of days when the character of Dementia took over, of course – snarling, paranoid, irrational – but those times usually came alongside illness or unhappiness. Perhaps it was a case of more delusions and increased loss of memory, but I really can't be sure. In fact, throughout the last of the days that we had together Mum was extremely *normal*. But that is the tragedy of dementia.

I have to think sometimes of Dr K. Did Mum have quality of life? he had asked. Put differently, did I do it right or at least right enough?

She had her favourite TV shows and videos. Her favourite TV chef was Huey. She loved Huey. He was a companion. *A Touch of Frost*, Inspector Frost, another companion. Amanda Burton in *Silent*

Witness. Greg Moore, the young tenor from *Scotland the Brave*. *The 7.30 Report*. Clarke and Dawe on Thursday nights. Steve Irwin on *Enough Rope*. The Lighthouse Family on *Parkinson*.

One Easter we watched *Jesus Christ Superstar* together. 'Was it a grand mistake?' I said when I was helping her to bed that night. 'Poor old Him!' She laughed at that. 'I've never heard Jesus described so before – "poor old Him"!'

We watched all the David Attenborough documentaries together. 'Mum, David's on!'

'Oh, David! Yes, of course. You can't mistake the voice,' she would say and then forget to listen.

I told her about his niece and members of her family dying in the tsunamis. 'We should write to him about that,' I said.

'Yes, we should write.'

We read books. Winston Graham's *Poldark*. Then Arthur Conan Doyle's *The Hound of the Baskervilles*. Patricia St John's *Star of Light*, set in the back streets of Morocco. We sat in the courtyard out back while she chopped privet and I read out Kipling's *Just So Stories* and *Mowgli*. We waded through Paul Burrell's *A Royal Duty* on his working life with Princess Diana. (Mum enjoyed it.) And we did most of the Laura Ingalls Wilder series. (She loved those.)

We had a simple life. We took pleasure in small things. Some things are commonplace, but no less valid. An opportunistic kookaburra came to the verandah one afternoon. We fed him cat food. She willed him back the next day and the day after, but he was gone. Another time I spotted a spider-eating wasp hauling a massive huntsman off towards her burrow. I called a nephew over and the three of us watched the wasp at her work – it seemed to take her forever before she had him hauled beyond our view.

When the moon was full I would take Mum out the front and we would gape at it as all people gape at the moon when they stop to contemplate it.

We spent a lot of time in the garden. Water use was restricted in those days so every Sunday and Wednesday night we watered the garden. I would move her in the wheelchair from one rose to the next. She still had projects. 'Are the secateurs there?' she would say. 'The geranium's getting a bit leggy.' In the winter we attacked the shrubs that needed pruning. One day the dog went mad and smashed to pieces the *Acanthus mollis* that grew by the back gate. Mum chopped off all the pulped leaves while I divided and replanted. There was always something to do in the garden.

The neighbours would come in sometimes for a cup of tea. Mrs Polden, Neville's wife, offered to sit with Mum sometimes to give me a break. And there were the checkout operators in the supermarket and Ra's friends. There were always kids and young adults about the place. In the last year Rock transformed our verandah/sunroom into a den. One night there was bash bash bash on the side door of the lounge room. 'It's Rock. Is it alright if me and my mates play poker out the back? We'll try and be quiet.' Mum went to bed, but she enjoyed having them out there.

And there were the outings. We took her to Old Government House for one birthday, Vaucluse House for another. We went to the Royal Easter Show all years. We went on the Rivercat once with Ra and Col from Meadowbank into the Quay. We wheeled her around the Botanic Gardens and then came back on the ferry. When Alexander turned eighteen the entire family met up for lunch at a restaurant in the Rocks and afterwards meandered down to the Harbour. (There's a photo somewhere.) There was ANZAC Day and the Community Transport trips – Parliament House, a picnic in Centennial Park, shopping at Birkenhead Point, the Fish Markets and our fortnightly sojourns to Carlingford Court.

She was still loved and still returned affection. She was still important and she knew it. Yes, Mum had quality of life.

Of course there are things that haunt us. The night she died Mum told one of the nurses that she knew she was dying and wanted to be home in her own bed. That haunts.

The stupid thing with the tablets haunts. She was *dying*. Why didn't I think to say leave off the unnecessary tablets? Leave off tablets altogether! Well, I just didn't think of it. The hospital was so busy that day and I just didn't think of it. All I was thinking was how to get her home so that she could watch Little House and die in the sanctity of her own bed.

I regret the unfulfilled promises I made, though there is no mileage in that either. One day we'll go into Town again. One day we'll get a taxi and go in to the Cathedral so you can go to church as you used to. One day. One day.

When I look back on those last three years, well I would do it all again tomorrow if I had the chance. I would change some things. I would not send her to the day centre because she really did not want to go. I hated sending her off like a little kid who didn't want to go to school. She would ask me to go with her. And she came home frustrated at being told what to do, 'pushed around', she called it. It took a while to calm her down after that and to get her 'back'. Once or twice she came home happy and relaxed. They had a therapy dog at the centre once. She talked about him all night. But that was about all. Others seem to genuinely enjoy the day centre, but Mum didn't – 'painting bloody rocks!' – so I should not have sent her. That was a mistake.

When it comes to looking after her, people tell me that I did the best I could. I don't think anybody ever really does that. But I tried. Mum died away from home in hospital, but even then we were with her. And she and I maintained our relationship to the end. We still argued and got impatient with each other. We still joked and shared affection. We maintained our relationship to the end.

'Fond of you, I am, Old Woman,' I would say.
'Fond of you, I am,' she would come back.
'That's lucky!'
'Luck has nothing to do with it.'
And she was right, of course. Luck had nothing to do with it.

Some useful contacts

Carer's Australia, <www.carersnsw.asn.au>, 1800 242 636 (business hours) or 1800 052 222 (emergency respite care)

Dementia Helpline, free call 1800 100 500

The Eldercare Forum – an American-based internet group that is very helpful for advice, information, inspiration and answers to specific queries, <http://eldercare.infopop.cc/6/ubb.x>

The Taxi Transport Subsidy Scheme offers half-price fares for disabled and frail aged people. Phone 1800 623 724 to access the form. The GP will have to fill in the medical details.

Bibliography

MedicineNet.com

<http://www.medicinenet.com/tacrine/article.htm>

Dementia Care Central

<http://www.dementiacarecentral.com/aboutdementia/treating/aricept>

Helpguide.com

<http://www.helpguide.org/elder/lewy_body_disease.htm>

Helpguide.org

<http://www.helpguide.org/elder/vascular_dementia.htm>

Department of Health and Ageing

<http://www.health.gov.au/internet/main/publishing.nsf/Content/ageing-dementia-stages/>

Australian Medical Association

<http://www.ama.com.au/node/264>

Sleep Disorders Australia

<http://www.sleepoz.org.au/>

Bryden, C., *Dancing with Dementia: My Story of Living Positively with Dementia*, Jessica Kingsley Publishers, 2005.

Connor, J., *A Funny Thing Happened on the Way to the Nursing Home*, Bookbound

Publishing, 1998.

Derkley, K., 'The Happier Home', *Good Weekend*, 4 September 2004.

Rain, M.S., *Love Never Sleeps: Living at Home with Alzheimer's*, Hampton Roads
Publishing Inc., Charlottesville, VA, 2002.

Sherry, J., 'Life Stories: Validating the Person', in *Australian Hospital & Healthcare*, p. 13, 2003.

Valenta, T., *Remember Me, Mrs V.? Caring for My Wife: Her Alzheimer's and Others' Stories*, Michelle Anderson Publishing, Melbourne, 2007.

Books on dementia

Jim Connor, *A Funny Thing Happened on the Way to the Nursing Home*

A Funny Thing Happened has a lot on delusions and the practicalities of caring. I did not always follow the method of going along with every delusion. But the book helped haul me out of my own gloom at an especially bad time when Mum was being combative and I was being combative back. *Believing* somebody goes a long way to calming down combativeness. Arguing and talking back only makes combativeness worse. It's a pointless endeavour.

Christine Bryden, *Dancing with Dementia: My Story of Living Positively with Dementia*

Christine Bryden has dementia. She has done a lot of advocacy work for people with dementia and writes and talks about the actual experience, how she deals with life now. She takes us into her reality.

Mary Summer Rain, *Love Never Sleeps: Living at Home with Alzheimer's*

Love Never Sleeps is not an easy read. There is an awful lot of personal material to wade through, most especially detail on family discord, which I felt overwhelmed the content and stated function of the book. Had I been given this book at the time I was caring for my own mother I would have had trouble getting through it. But I have since read the book and I found myself thinking often what I would have done in situations the carers found themselves in. And that is, after all, the reason why we write about caring and dementia.

Tom Valenta, *Remember Me, Mrs V.?*

Tom Valenta's wife, Marie, was fifty-four when she was diagnosed with Alzheimer's disease. The Valentas have also done a lot of public work for people with dementia. *Remember Me, Mrs V.?* does not deal with the day to day nuts and bolts of caring, but explores the medical and social impacts of life with dementia.